Chunging

The Cleansing Side of Medicine

by Yunjo Chung, M.D.

Mosaic Press
Cincinnati

Painting on cover by Myung-jin Chung

Yosemite Series, No. Thirteen
33" X 40" Acrylic and mixed media

Book Illustrations by Dianne Johnson

Photo by Barbara J. Gottling

ISBN 0-88014-084-4

Library of Congress Catalog Card Number
91-062319

Distributed by:

Cincinnati OB-GYN, Inc.
5889 Colerain Avenue, Cincinnati, Ohio 45239
513-923-4018 FAX 513-923-4301
800-255-6476 yjchung1@msn.com

Mosaic Press
Cincinnati

Acknowledgments

First of all, I thank my beloved wife, the artist Myung-jin. Without her, nothing in my life would have been possible the past thirty-three years.

Like many Western physicians, I used to believe that miracle drugs would eventually conquer all human illness. When I, myself, was inflicted with sickness, I took the appropriate medicines and got better. However, I soon began suffering from severe side effects caused by the very drugs which had helped me.

I want to thank Moon-jo Chung, Ph.D., a prominent chemist, who taught me a proper breathing method during this period of illness and re- introduced me to slow exercises which I had often seen performed when I was a child in Korea. Following this regimen, I became healthier than before I was ill.

With this personal experience as a beginning, I have refined this method over the years, and continue to be rejuvenated. I have tried to determine the factual basis for this, and to form theories as to why these simple behavior changes could make such a miraculous change in my health and in the health of many of my patients.

I want to thank William B. Chung, M.D., my youngest son, who drafted a note of my thoughts and findings for me to present to a publisher.

I was fortunate to find Miriam Owen Irwin, publisher of Mosaic Press books, who had the open mind to listen and the ability to understand. I especially thank Miriam, who edited this book herself, for her courage and perseverance in publishing this book in spite of her own personal difficulties. I greatly appreciate also the wisdom and input of her husband, Ken Irwin, whose background in physiology and chemistry helped me to define the overall picture of what I was trying to say. Thanks also to Jay Erisman for both his excellent literary editing and skillful scientific proofreading.

I sincerely thank Ivan Tuskan, M.D., Paul J. Haas, M.D., and Gale W. Miller, M.D., for their encouragement and support

Finally, I want to thank my other two sons, Jeff B. Chung, M.D. and Michael B. Chung, M.D., with whom I constantly discussed this work as I was forming the logic of my thoughts.

Y.C.

July 26, 1996

Table of Contents

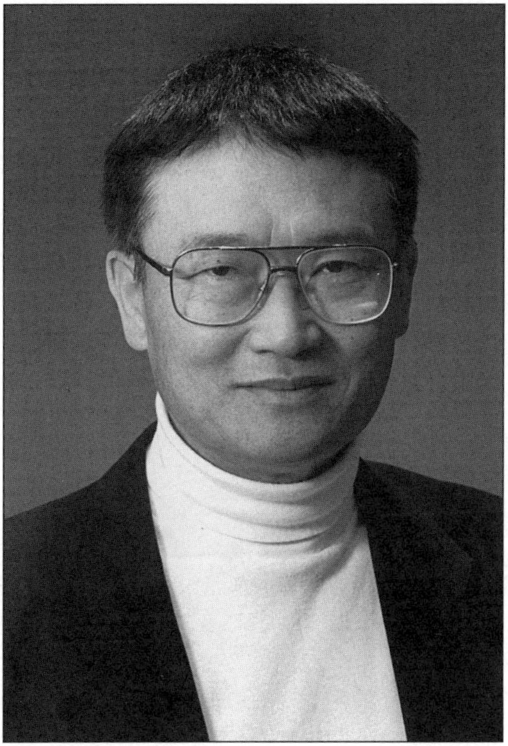

Yunjo Chung, M.D.

Dr. Chung was educated in Korea, completing his M.D. in 1963 from the University of Korea. He came to the United States for further medical training in 1966. He is Board certified in Obstetrics and Gynecology since 1973. By that time, he had fallen in love with America, and he and his wife became citizens of the United States. He wants to contribute to the betterment of his beloved adopted country by teaching people to cleanse away the cause of disease to prevent and cure illness and to keep them functionally fit their whole lives.

PLEASE
READ THIS BOOK
FROM BEGINNING TO END

Dr. Chung builds his ideas so carefully, one step at a time, that if you miss one part, ideas he presents further on in the book may not be as meaningful to you.

Please don't skip around—don't ignore a chapter because you think that subject doesn't apply to you, or because you already know a lot about that topic.

Undoubtedly you already know lots and lots of health facts. But its *the understanding* of what all those facts really mean as a whole health system which Dr. Chung has presented here which is so wonderful, so promising of a better life—both for you as an individual and for us all as a society.

Miriam Owen Irwin
Publisher

Where is the Fountain of Youth?

There is a well-known Korean legend about an emperor. He had power and influence, wealth, women. Anything at all that he wanted, he could have. But that was not enough for him. He wanted more. The Emperor wanted to live forever.

The Emperor sent thousands of men all over the world to find something, *anything*, which would make him younger. His subjects searched everywhere. After years of seeking, a travel-weary nobleman brought him a Root of Long Life.

That was the famous naturally grown mountain ginseng root. Found deep in the mountains in Korea, mountain ginseng lives for hundreds of years. It was believed that mountain ginseng could cure all human disease and lengthen human life. This belief had gone unchallenged until Western logic and research found out that the major effect of the ginseng root was a placebo effect. That is, it appeared to work because people *believed* it would work.

This longing for eternal life is not limited to Asia. In almost all cultures, there are substances thought to extend life or to miraculously improve health. Horn of young deer has been used as a natural life extender. The gall bladder of the bear has been used as a cure-all for many diseases. The penis and testicles of the seal have been used as a male potency drug. All these ancient 'remedies' were extremely expensive, and according to double-blind scientific research (a respected and often-used form of research), they were effective only because people had faith that they would work.

The remedies I have mentioned are all harmless to humans. Unfortunately, this is not always the case. Historically, many toxic substances were believed to have curative properties.

At the turn of this century, it was widely thought that tiny doses of arsenic made ladies have lovely white skin. Years ago, my publisher's grandmother told her that when she was young, all her girlfriends had taken small doses of arsenic continuously, but she had never taken any. "It did give them a beautiful pale look," she said. "But they are all dead now."

Besides arsenic, various other chemicals including mercury and sulphur were added to 'health elixirs' which usually had an alcohol base. Some were mostly alcohol, and many a temperance leader gulped down certain tonics because the drugs *did* make them feel better—for a little while.

Use of these remedies was not confined to the lay public. Well-respected physicians believed in certain medicines and prescribed them for their patients. 'Health elixirs' were given to kings and queens by doctors with only good intentions at heart. Historically, many members of the royalty died young.

When modern researchers investigated their deaths, it was found that many of these ancient kings died of poisoning.

Today, we laugh at these archaic practices and dismiss them as out-of-date. Unfortunately, we still fall prey to the same type of medical misconceptions. At any pharmacy or health food store you will find shelves full of 'natural vitamins' that contain all sorts of plant roots and other 'ancient remedies'. The purveyors of these natural vitamins claim that this product will make your skin look young, or that concoction will make your hair shine. *Do not be fooled.* In the majority of cases, any beneficial effects of these natural vitamins come from convincing the patient to *think* that they will work. If you believe a thing will work, it just might. If you think it won't work, it probably won't.

We are a youth-conscious society. We are bombarded with the media's message that we need to appear young: "you must look young to be attractive, and to look young, you must buy this product." Even the medical community has been affected by this media-induced drive.

Recently, in the *New England Journal of Medicine*, an article was published concerning the youth-enhancing effects of a naturally occurring substance called 'human growth hormone' (HGH). The article stated that this hormone, for the measly cost of $14,000 per year, could make a person look and feel twenty years younger by building muscle, thinning fat, and tightening the skin. According to the author of the article, people using this hormone feel healthy and energetic. However, the article did not say that HGH would make people live longer or be less susceptible to disease. Instead, the article mentioned that prolonged usage of HGH could cause heart failure, diabetes, high blood pressure, and other damaging side effects. In time, HGH may prove to be just another false hope, one more drug that did not live up to its hype.

The very best that all these external sources of 'youth' might accomplish is to give the *appearance* of youth without actual youth. In fact, like many of the ancient remedies before them, they may actually shorten life.

In reality, many people are afraid of longevity of life. When people think of a chronological old age, images of nursing homes, medicine, loneliness, and pain come to mind. This type of suffering is unnatural and unnecessary.

I believe a person can be fully functional until the moment of death. This type of natural death occurs often in the animal kingdom; wild animals, reaching the point of death, simply walk away and die peacefully. Animals don't go in for all the foolishness we go through in trying to recapture the fleeting look of youth. Humans comb the planet in their search for a fountain of youth; they look for it in herbs, in balms, creams, pills, elixirs. One food after another is popular as the current health fad. One company after another makes a fortune selling these products. Most things that won't hurt you, won't help you either. But still we try—still we continue to search for something wonderful outside ourselves that we can swallow, sip, or rub on our skin.

Fully functional long life should be our goal, not just to look young. *The fountain of youth lies within yourself.* The ability to stay young lies within your own mind and your own body, and you must search there, and nowhere else.

Chunger vs. Younger

People believe that every day after you are born you get older and closer to death.

That is generally true—but many of my patients have made themselves more physically functional with every day by following my directions and exercises. I have actually witnessed my patients lengthening their lives at the same time they improve the quality of their life.

For example, Ms. Sandra T. was a fifty-five year old executive of a small company. She was five feet three inches tall, weighed 190 pounds, and had a blood pressure of 160/95. (The upper limit of normal pressure is 140/90.) She regularly took in an excessive amount of caffeine, salt, and alcohol, and never exercised. One day, Sandra took an employee who had suffered minor injuries to the emergency room. She was agitated at having to be at the hospital and away from work. Suddenly, Sandra began to experience severe chest pain and fell unconscious; she had a heart attack. If she had not been in the emergency room at the time, she would have died.

As she recovered, Sandra began to realize the importance of proper diet and exercise. One year after this incident, her weight had dropped to 130 pounds, the weight she was when she was 30 years old. Her blood pressure had dropped to 130/80. Her doctors told her that she could look forward to a normal life expectancy and be fully functional if she stuck to her new-found good behavior of proper diet and exercise.

Aging is the whole body illness. People who have a positive attitude toward illness like "I am too healthy to catch flu," find that they rarely do get flu. If they do come down with flu, they recover more quickly because they have the attitude, "I will get better very quickly because I am very healthy."

It surprises me that people who have such a positive attitude toward life often have a pessimistic attitude toward aging. They say, "Don't fight against aging. Age graciously."

During their entire lives, people often see that a positive attitude can change any situation in their favor. So why do they give up when it comes to aging? I think one reason people give up is because there are no positive words to help them fight aging. People cannot cling to a concept of getting younger while aging only because there is no word describing that condition. The only words they know are negative, such as "I am getting older" and "I cannot get younger." The opposite idea would be to say "I am not getting older" and "I am getting younger." However, these positive words, "I am getting younger," are logically impossible to a thinking person. Everyone knows you don't actually get younger.

I have searched for a word in English which represents the process of becoming more mentally and emotionally fit and more physically functional. In English, as there is presently no word for this concept, I have a new word: 'Chunger' (pronounced *chun' ger*). This word means "becoming emotionally and physically healthier as time passes." A Chunger person is functionally fit.

That is why it is so important to use the phrase "I am getting Chunger as I get older". With the idea of this new and logical word, 'Chunger', engraved in your mind, the *concept* allows you to develop a positive attitude to fight against aging, the whole-body disease.

The Chinese word 正 (pronounced *chung*) means right against wrong, good against evil, honest against dishonest, correct against incorrect, proper against improper, healthy against diseased, and normal against abnormal.

But how do you become physically and mentally healthier? You can do this by 'Chunging'. Chunging is any act of exercise, breathing, diet, or positive attitude which makes a person get Chunger. Chunging is natural and easy. Any exercise which could hurt a person is not a Chunging exercise. An exercise which cannot hurt a person, but which can only make him or her healthier, is a Chunging exercise.

For example, running is not Chunging for people over the age of forty. When people over age forty start running regularly, more than ninety percent of them cannot continue to run because of a minor injury like a sprained ankle, or a major problem such as a broken knee joint or a heart attack.

To me, it seems that the odds of getting healthier by running are no better than the odds of getting rich by gambling.

It is ridiculous for a person to start running for better health and then end up with broken cartilage in the knee. Of course, statistically speaking, out of 1,000 runners, there should be a few who get healthier. But I hate to think of the unnecessary pain, inconvenience, and expense of the injuries all the others receive from that jarring exercise.

Again, a Chunging diet is very different from an ordinary weight reduction diet. People who lose weight by a diet pill or commercial diet usually find that the loss is temporary. Most gain back all the weight they lost—and gain more.

With the Chunging diet, you lose weight much more slowly until you reach your healthy weight, but you should never gain it back again. It takes much longer—Chunging is *not* a "get-the-pounds-off-fast" kind of diet. But doesn't a plan which gives you the ability to maintain your weight, once you have achieved the loss, seem like a better idea?

The principal of Chunging is derived from the basic Chinese philosophy of medicine: the theory of *ki* (pronounced *key*).

The theory of *ki* is based on the following ideas:

1. When *ki* in a person flows well in the whole body, then he or she is healthy. When it flows poorly, the patient is sick.

2. When *ki* does not flow well (or is blocked) in certain organs of the human body, those organs eventually become diseased. If you can make the *ki* flow well again by drugs, acupuncture, or by applying heat and massage, you can cure the disease.

I have heard that the ancients came by this wisdom through watching the Yellow River. This river flows through China and is notorious for frequent devastating floods throughout its history. There was a saying that those who are able to control the Yellow River can rule the universe.

Dynasties rose and fell along with the fate of the Yellow River. Many emperors tried to protect their subjects from the floods by building dikes and levees. After a few thousand years of repeated failures of trying to control the river by blocking it with dikes, they finally learned that it could not be controlled unless they made the angry water flow out at about the same rate as it flows in.

Such a simple, common sense solution. A large amount of water comes in and the same amount of water has to go out. Intake and output has to be balanced. If you block the flow it will overrun. Do not block the flow. Let it flow. Let it flow.

In ancient China, doctors applied this principle to the human body. Humans have to take clean *ki* (energy from nutrients) into the body, let *ki* flow well in the body (metabolism), then let dirty *ki* out of the body (expelling the waste). When this energy-flow mechanism runs smoothly, there is health. If *ki* is not flowing smoothly, it means the waste is still somewhere in the body. If it is in the body, it is in the body's cells, poisoning them, making them more susceptible to disease.

Today's doctors, researchers, and food and drug industries are concentrating on producing better nutrients and drugs and more refreshing liquids. They are always prescribing one new thing or another for the purpose of achieving better health. I often think it is their own financial health that worries them.

Modern medicine almost totally neglects the expulsion of the end products, which is just as important as the intake of nutrients and drugs. There has long been a belief that nature will expel whatever junk you put into a body. This is just like the earlier days when industries dumped their toxic waste into the rivers with the belief that nature would take care of the toxins. We now know this isn't necessarily true.

To keep the cell healthy and disease-free, the output is more important than the intake. If the output is shut off, the cell will get sick, even if you give it the best nutrients, miracle drugs, or pure oxygen. If the output flows freely, the cell will quickly expel waste, even if it ingests a little toxic material.

The main purpose and result of Chunging is the proper cleansing of living body cells by expelling waste, carbon dioxide, and contaminated water.

Please read this book from beginning to end. If you jump around only to the chapters that interest you, you may miss a true understanding of the basic philosophy of Chunging. I have tried to present the ideas step by step so that the understanding of one chapter is dependent upon the text before.

The Purpose of Exercise

It is obvious that the object of exercise is to make a person healthier. However, so many people become unhealthy directly or indirectly as a result of so-called exercises that a new medical field has developed because millions of people have become injured while exercising. That field is called sports medicine, and physicians in that field earn tons of money.

How ironic! Exercising to get healthier, only to end up crippled or injured. Chunging exercises are never jarring or violent exercises. Chunging *will* make you healthier, and more energetic—but you must follow the directions carefully. Chunging exercises can and should be continued into old age. At any age, your joints will become more flexible, your muscles will be toned up, you will be able to think more clearly, and you will look and feel rejuvenated.

How does Chunging achieve these miracles? Chunging exercises are designed to accomplish the following:

1. Improve blood circulation to organs, tissues, and cells by gentle exercising and rubbing.

2. Improve metabolism by increasing oxygenation both through proper breathing and by working the muscles.

3. Eliminate all body waste and contaminants by drinking more water and by proper breathing.

What does all this do? It cleans your body and its organs by cleansing the individual cells. Chunging exercises rejuvenate you by cleansing your body of waste on the cellular level.

Any exercise which makes you feel tired may be harmful to you. Tiredness is evidence of unnecessary accumulation of body wastes and microscopic injuries on a cellular level. Any exercise that causes more than moderate shortness of breath may harm you by inducing anaerobic metabolism in your body. This is called oxygen debt. If you experience shortness of breath after exercise, it is evidence of a lack of oxygen.

The Chunging Exercise

If you want to know what is the most important exercise for humans, you must observe human infants. The human infant's first and most important act is breathing. This is vital to life itself.

As soon as the newborn is breathing, he starts moving all the joints he has. This is the second physical exercise humans perform. It is important because a joint cannot stay healthy unless it moves constantly through its whole range of motion. The infant also cries, sucks, urinates, and defecates.

Once an infant masters coordination of movement, then he learns to sit up from a lying-down position. This is the third most important exercise. Fourth, the infant learns to stand up from a sitting position.

After an infant has mastered these four essential physical activities, which usually takes a year, he then starts walking, running, and jumping. Running and jumping are the last and least important as well as the most dangerous movements.

No one would try to make an infant, who was having a difficult time sitting up, try to master running and jumping because it is very likely that the child would be too weak and would suffer injuries.

Ironically, there are many exercise instructors who encourage an adult to run or to jump around even if he has a difficult time sitting up from a lying position. For example, a middle-aged woman goes to a new aerobics class. As she is on her feet when she goes in, she joins the class and jumps around, following the lithe instructor who has been doing this every day. This same woman cannot sit up from a prone position without using her arms nor can she get out of a chair without pulling herself up. Within a week, she has to drop out of the class due to an injury.

Consider the man in his late thirties with a sedentary job who decides he will join some friends for racquetball. If he hasn't run or participated in sports for years, he is in danger of injury.

The violent exercises which are now popular frequently induce joint and back pain due to injuries received while exercising. What young, athletic people can do in exercises shown on television has nothing at all to do with what most people *should* do.

No matter what your age, to maintain a functional life, adults should be able to perform all of these basic-to-life exercises: sitting, standing, bending, and squatting.

As incredibly important as these simple movements are, many adults give up some of these basic movements over the years through lack of exercise.

Any period of inactivity, such as inactivity due to illness, may decrease a person's ability to perform. Also, people who exert themselves following surgery, often break out in a cold sweat. They get alarmed and stop exerting. A couple of weeks later, when they have healed, they do not start to exercise again. Actually, this is one of the main ways people *appear* to have aged—their friends say, "That illness took a lot out of him", or "She was never the woman she was before the operation".

If they do not actively work at "getting back in shape" as soon as the illness or injury is over, they may be unable to perform some of these essential movements for the rest of their lives:

- Many people cannot sit up from a lying position without using their hands and arms. Stomach and back muscles should be doing this work.

- Many older people cannot get out of a chair without pulling themselves up with their arms. They should be using their thigh muscles.

- Most older people bend at the waist when they pick up something from the floor. By doing this for years, they can no longer do deep knee bends. Their big thigh muscles need to be stretched and rebuilt.

- Sitting down on the floor and getting up again is difficult for most older people.

These are all absolutely basic to functional life! Chunging exercises will give you back these basic movements and improve your range of motion. Chunging exercises are designed to slowly and gently stretch muscles and flex joints.

Just because you can't do what you once could, does not mean that you cannot regain that ability. You can!

Stiff joints *will* move easily again. You will retain mobility and full functional use of your body as long as you live.

Fully Functional Cells

A human body is composed of approximately 100 trillion living cells. If you keep your cells young, you will stay young. Your cells *have* the power to get Chunger. How do you tap the power of youth? Simply let your cells live normal lives.

Then what is a normal life for a cell? Cells are just like you. After they are formed, they may live a peaceful, useful life, or terrible things might happen to them through injury or by exposure to toxic substances. They may be injured and be unable to function well.

To sustain your life:

1. The cells must absorb nutrients and oxygen.

2. The cells must perform their specific work.

3. The cells must be able to expel the waste.

In other words, cells must eat, work, and poop.

If enough of your cells aren't working perfectly, you will surely feel it in some way. You are, after all, the sum of all those trillions of cells.

Humans have concentrated on production, marketing, distribution of goods. No one gave much thought to the accumulation of waste until the earth was in danger of dying due to our mountains of garbage. Pollution from waste is poisoning our world, possibly making it uninhabitable.

When human beings find the way to properly eliminate this garbage, the earth will revive quickly. The same thing is true in your body. If you could learn how to eliminate the waste on a cellular level, rather than to concentrate on what you take in, you could begin to rejuvenate your body today.

The main source of disease and aging is the accumulation of body waste. It is cellular waste that produces dysfunction of the cells. When their vital structures become damaged or when waste is present and persists, individual cells become diseased as their power to fight against germs is hindered.

Therefore, it is not only germs to blame when illness strikes—everyone knows a 'run down' person gets sick easily. What this really means is that many of the exhausted person's individual cells have accumulated waste to the point that they are not able to effectively fight the invading bacteria.

Past and present medicine has concentrated on finding the miracle drug to overcome the disease, not on eliminating the cause of disease. Most drugs, even those with beneficial action for one organ or part of the body, are just another harmful chemical to the rest of your body's individual cells.

Even at this moment, most scientists and doctors concentrate on nutrition. A few study metabolism, but very few are researching the importance of excretion, let alone excretion at the cellular level.

When something is rotten in your kitchen and producing foul odors, using deodorizing sprays and bug killer is not the answer. Taking out the garbage is the correct solution.

The key to rejuvenating your body is proper cleansing of your body's living cells. Elimination of cellular waste is the most important factor in staying fully functional into old age.

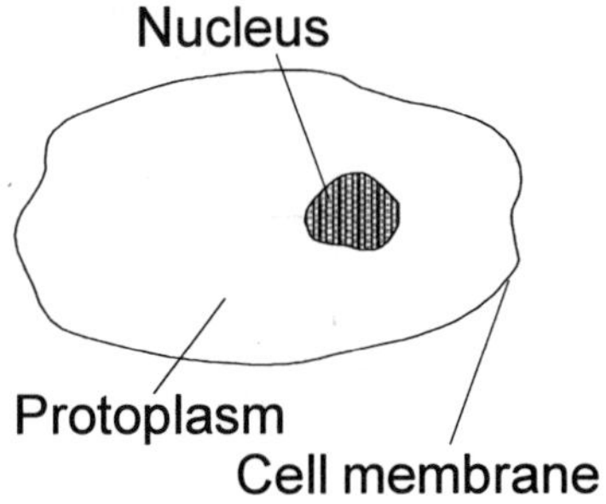

Fifty years ago this simplistic view of the cell was taught in high school science; a cell has a nucleus floating in a jelly-like substance covered by a bubble-like membrane.

Now we know that cells are much more complex. Each one contains a chemical factory capable of producing different compounds. But not all cells produce the same chemicals.

Did you know that cells can get constipated? They can. Cells can also get indigestion. Sometimes cells get tired. They can get thirsty and hungry. They are formed from a parent cell, they live, they work and they die. Cells are just like you!

Due to what we have learned from electron microscopes, the following two pages show a simplified, updated idea of some of the structures we can now see now 'see' inside a cell:

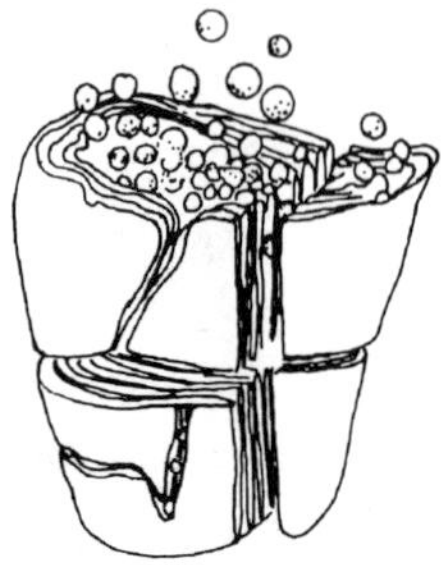

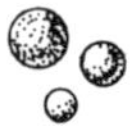

Secretion granules are produced by the Golgi apparatus.

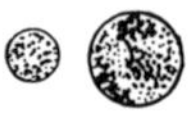

Lysosomes digest foreign matter in the cell, and are thought to be produced by the Golgi apparatus.

The Golgi apparatus governs the secretory functions of the cell and stores proteins until they are needed.

Centrioles help organize the chromosomes during cell division.

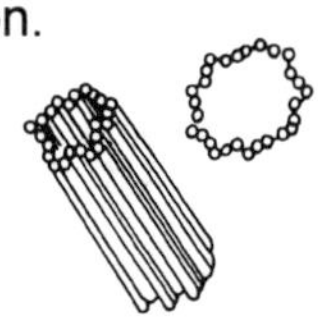

The hard working cell membrane is extremely complex. It can allow certain substances in or keep them out as directed by commands from hormones. (For example, the hormone insulin forces sugar out of the blood stream and through the membrane of individual cells.) The membrane also has a protein coating which helps it fend off attacks from bacteria and viruses or foreign substances.

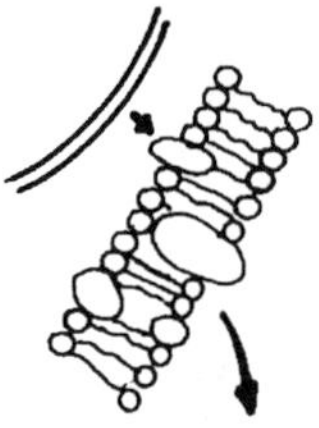

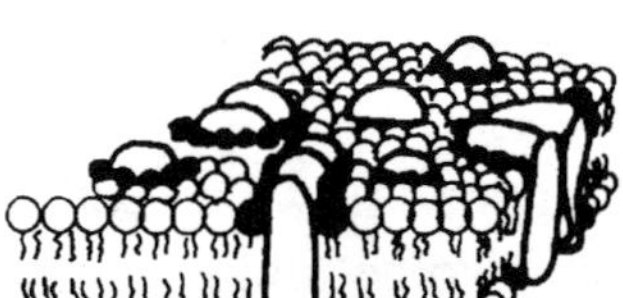

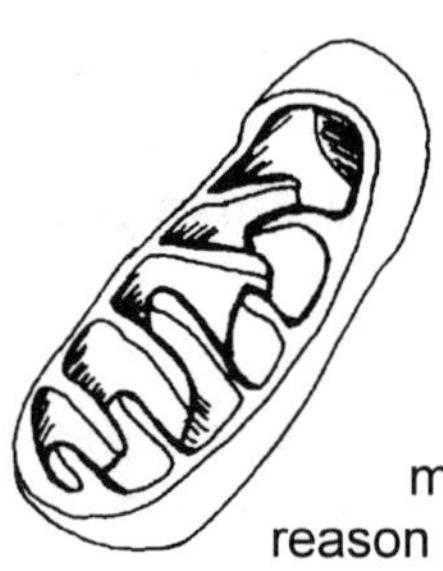

Mitochondria are the body's energy factories. Healthy cells make more mitrochondria when more are needed, a major reason why people who exercise have more energy.

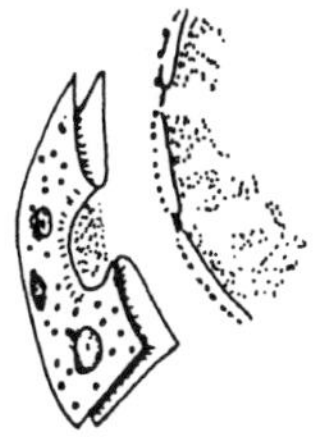

The nuclear envelope encloses the nucleus.

The nucleus (not pictured here) is the 'brain' of the cell—the president, auditor, factory manager, and when necessary, the cell's executioner. The nucleus of each cell contains perfect copies of the body's unique chromosomes.

Among the contents of the nucleus is the nucleolus (below), which helps produce ribosomes.

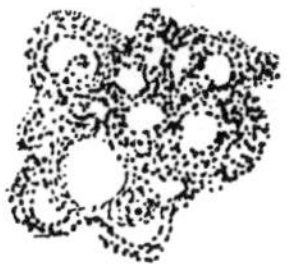

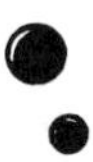

Lipid droplets temporarily store fat for future consumption.

Ribosomes (not pictured), which produce proteins, are attached to the endoplasmic reticulum, and are so small that even under an electron microscope, they appear only as dots.

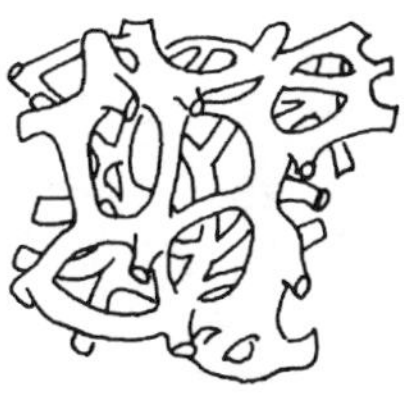

Smooth reticulum

Endoplasmic reticulum provides pathways for the transport of chemicals within the cell plasma.

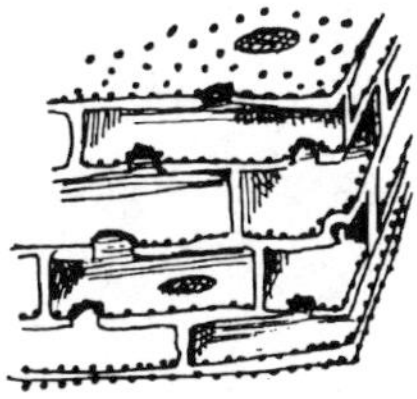

Rough reticulum

These diagrams show just a few of the many incredible structures we now know are inside a cell. They are each 'doing their thing'—living, working, consuming nutrients and oxygen, producing waste.

Electron microscopes took their first pictures in 1945; since then they have been steadily improved. They can now magnify 100,000 times.

Because of these great scientific improvements, we now know much more about the interior of the cell than we did even a few years ago.

There are many more parts within a cell than we thought there were, and recently, we've realized that each component is extremely complicated. The cell membrane itself is an incredibly complex structure which performs many tasks.

I hope you can begin to appreciate your body's amazing and wonderful structure—and I certainly hope you see the need to take better care of yourself on a cellular level.

A fully functional person has fully functional cells. You *should and you can* accomplish this by Chunging exercises and by following good Chunging practices.

A Gynecologist's Observations

After spending four years in medical school, surviving the stench of anatomy lab, treating street people in the emergency room as an intern, serving as a medical officer in the Navy for three years, and after a four year OB-GYN residency, I thought I had smelled a good cross-section of the human race.

When my residency was finally over, I joined an established OB-GYN group practice with patients from middle- and upper-class families.

One of the most difficult parts of my practice is, with certain individuals, to endure an offensive vaginal odor while I was thoroughly examining my patient's genitals. Some women smell terrible! Twice, after such examinations, I actually went to the bathroom and vomited.

Sometimes, a patient's offensive body odor requires my nurses to use deodorizing sprays to air out the room when the patient leaves. The odor can be so pervasive and lingering that we simply have to close up the room for the rest of the day.

Odor might be expected on grossly overweight women unless they take great pains to be fastidious. A street person who rarely bathes can reasonably be expected to stink.

However, in my OB-GYN practice, I was dealing with well-groomed, neat-looking women. They had money to spend on clothes, cosmetics, soaps, and feminine hygiene supplies. They came from homes which afforded them both the time and the privacy to take care of themselves. None of them were ignorant women. And none of the cases of offensive body odor were caused by any apparent serious medical problem.

Very few of my patients had this objectionable odor, but I considered it very serious for the ones who did. I decided that such a nauseating odor could not be natural. Clean healthy people just don't smell that bad. I found myself thinking about body odor. I decided to study and observe.

These intelligent, beautiful women did only normally accepted things to their bodies. Bathing, douching, powdering, perfuming, and using deodorants are all ordinary, common, run-of-the mill activities for a large proportion of the American female population. All of these things are supposed to eliminate body odor or cover it up. These chemical products have long been accepted by society.

And yet, *in spite of all their efforts,* these women had strong, unpleasant body odor. After thinking more about it, this treatment of their bodies struck me as very unnatural and possibly harmful. I began to think about the problem from the point of view of individual cells. How did all these things the women were doing affect ordinary skin cells?

History of a Case of Vaginal Odor

Through my experience as a gynecologist, I discovered why some people have little body odor while others have a lot. In order to share these ideas with you, I will take you through the case study of Mary G.

Mary G. is thirty-two years old, 130 pounds, and stands five foot eight inches tall. She is a middle-class, divorced elementary school teacher who had been suffering from recurrent vaginal infection, odor, and discharge for the last seven years. She was first treated by her family physician, then by a local gynecologist, and finally by a gynecology professor from a local medical university. After each treatment of vaginal suppositories, vaginal creams, and oral medicines, her symptoms began to fade. However, after she stopped taking the medicine, her symptoms would return.

Mary G. is a very 'clean' person. She appears neat, and with the help of some perfume, has a pleasant odor. She takes a shower every morning with soap and water and even takes a bubble bath before she goes to bed. Mary also douches after each menstrual period and occasionally after having sex. She wears silk or cotton-crotched nylon underwear. As you can see, her behavior seems very 'clean.' The odor became noticeable only when she took off her clothes.

On the recommendation of her friend, Mary decided to come see me. On examination of Mary's genitals, I noticed that her labia minor and labia major were reddish in color. This color indicates inflammation of the genital skin. She also had a foul vaginal odor. These findings, along with her yellow-white cottage cheese-like vaginal discharge are typical findings for a yeast infection. Examination of this discharge under the microscope confirmed this diagnosis as *vaginal candidiasis*, a yeast infection. However, yeast infections alone do not carry such a foul odor.

She had been treated for the yeast infection by many doctors, but the foul odor never left. The symptoms of yeast infection always soon returned.

If the odor wasn't caused by the vaginitis, it was caused by something else. She was working so hard at cleaning her genitals that she damaged her body's natural protection. After I treated and instructed Mary, her symptoms disappeared in three days. In three weeks, her disease was cured. In the last three years, she has had no recurrent infections and no vaginal odor. She has remarried and now has one healthy child.

There are millions of women like Mary in the U.S. who suffer from frequent or recurrent vaginitis, vaginal discharge, and vaginal odor. Ninety percent of all these women can be permanently cured of vaginal odor if they understand and follow my instructions.

How to Cure Vaginitis

So many of my patients were *too* clean. They were taking so many showers and baths, and using so much junk on their skin trying to be even cleaner, inside and out, that they were destroying their skin's own natural protection and damaging the delicate vaginal epithelium, the vaginal skin cells.

The same thing was true about vaginitis. Healthy women, once they realized they had a little vaginal discharge, felt dirty, and tried everything they could to eliminate the problem. They bathed, douched, used more over-the-counter products, which, after all, are chemicals. More times than not, the condition was aggravated.

I started advising those patients with a mild case of vaginitis, and who had no other gynecological problems, to stop douching, stop using soap to wash their genitals, and to wash with water only. I suggested they wear only cotton underwear to stay cooler and dryer. The wearing of silk or nylon panties causes greater collection of moisture which nurtures germ growth.

The typical reaction of the patients who followed my instructions is that for the first three weeks, the patient would feel so dirty and smelly that she would be afraid to walk in public because she thought other people could smell her foul odor. She was also afraid to have sexual contact with her husband because of this odor.

However, after the first three weeks, the patient would begin to notice that her genitals did not smell as bad as they had before she stopped using soap. She would soon realize that she noticed less lingering odor on her clothes when she took them off. She felt that her odor was receding and would report to me that her genitals felt cleaner. After three months, the patient felt that she was one hundred peercent better.

In fact, many of my patients told me that after six months of no soaping and no douching, their husbands would actually tell them how good they smelled.

The Clean Vagina

A clean vagina is the cleanest thing there is. Nature planned it that way. Nature provided a built-in method of natural protection to provide a clean environment for child-bearing, and to fight against infection.

This natural protection is a type of good bacteria called *Doedelein bacillus,* which lives inside the vagina. This helpful bacteria protects the female genitals from harmful germs by producing an acidic environment inside the vagina. This acidic environment helps eliminate any harmful germs while remaining harmless to the vagina itself. The actions of *Doedelein bacillus* help to keep the vagina clean.

The vagina is located very close to the anus where a wide variety of germs reside. It is very simple for these germs to travel into the vagina. Without the protection of the *Doedelein bacillus*, these germs will multiply and infect the vagina, causing the vagina to have an unpleasant odor.

Thus it is extremely important that the vagina remain very clean, which is only possible through the acid-producing action of the beneficial *Doedelein bacillus.*

Abdominal internal organs are located inside the peritoneal cavity. This cavity is 'germ free'; it has no disease-causing germs present. If germs are introduced into this cavity, an infection called peritonitis spreads very quickly. This infection is extremely harmful and can even cause death. If harmful germs travel even as far as the Fallopian tubes, they will cause inflammatory disease and abscesses which can cause scarring of the tubes which in turn can lead to infertility, even after treatment with antibiotics.

Please study the following picture. You will see there is a path through the uterus and fallopian tubes which is not sealed off from the interior of the body.

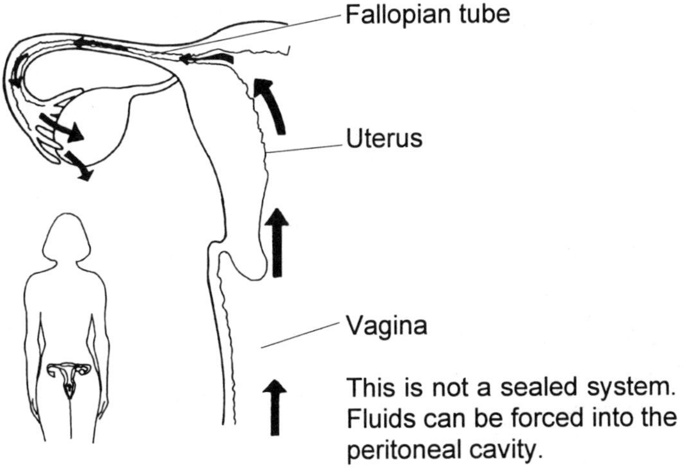

If water or air is forced into the vagina under pressure, as in douching, it is possible that air or water will travel through the uterine cavity and Fallopian tubes into the peritoneal cavity. Also, during intercourse, the piston-like action of the penis inside the vagina may force the contents of the vagina (such as fluid, air, germs, and sperm) into the peritoneal cavity.

More than twenty years ago, researchers concluded that douching can only harm the body and increase the likelihood of disease. Why then do women continue to douche when most gynecologists tell them not to? Probably for some of the same reasons people still smoke cigarettes after smoking has been proven to be harmful. They douche because other women do it and because commercials brainwash them by telling them that douching will make them clean and 'fresh', another favorite word of the ad agencies. Many healthy women douche because of a small amount of vaginal discharge and/or odor, which comes right back a day or two after douching.

If they douche, they are washing away their natural protection. If these women would simply try *not* douching for three weeks, to allow time for the good bacteria to re-create the normal acidic condition in the vagina, they may find that the vaginal discharge is diminished and that unpleasant odor is no longer a problem.

Normal vaginal discharge is creamy in color with a mucous consistency. It may have slight, but not a foul odor.

Any discharge which has a greenish or deep yellow color would be a sign to see your physician immediately. There is no reason at all to be shy or hesitant about consulting your doctor about any vaginal problem. Not seeking treatment immediately when you have a problem is the dumbest thing you can do. Almost all conditions are easily cured.

Again, remember, neither male nor female genitals should smell offensive. A healthy odor should be attractive to the opposite sex.

Let's Begin with Skin

One afternoon, a new patient came to see me who appeared to be about thirty years old. Her skin had no defects, not even dryness. On examination, I noticed that her genitals were healthy and carried no odor. When I looked at her chart, I was surprised to discover that she was fifty years old—not thirty, as I had thought.

I suspected, since she had no genital odor, that she was not using soap or douching. I asked her whether she washed with soap. She appeared to be very embarrassed and asked me, "Do I smell that bad?"

I laughed, and told her, "No. Because you have *no smell,* and your genitals appear to be so clean, I know that you could not be douching or using soap to wash your genitals. You are doing exactly the right thing. Continue to wash not using soap and not douching." I asked her how she learned to avoid the use of soap.

She told me that her mother, a nurse who emigrated from Europe, told her not to use soap, not only on her genitals, but on her entire body. I was amazed. She then told me that, although she felt she was clean, she always worried that someone would discover that she was not using soap and accuse her of being 'dirty'.

I asked her, "How do you wash?" She told me that she washed in water only. I asked her if she used a washcloth. She replied that she rubbed her skin only with her hands as she washed.

Thinking about this case made me begin to suspect that using soap may have a detrimental effect on skin aging. It was already well known that smoking and sun had adverse effects on skin. Perhaps using soap is as hard on the rest of a person's skin as it is on the delicate tissue of the genitals.

After this, I began to ask my patients how they washed their bodies. From these inquiries, this is what I have come to believe:

- People who use little or no soap on their face have fewer wrinkles and less acne.
- People who use less soap on their bodies have less skin disease, such as moles, rashes, eczema, and skin psoriasis.
- People who use no soap on their genital and anal areas have less vaginitis, less vaginal odor, fewer hemorrhoids.

Americans are *obsessed* with cleanliness. We want to look clean, smell clean, feel clean. We are flooded with advertising hype for personal hygiene products, and we respond by spending a lot of money on these products.

Let's Burst Soap's Bubble

Americans know how to make things 'clean'. Just wash with soap and water, they believe, because they know that soap can clean your body, your car, your dishes, and more. This is what they have been taught all their lives.

Soap. What a beautiful gift to humanity! *Is it really?*

The advertising spiel goes like this: Soap kills germs. Since it kills germs, there can be no disease. Soap makes you clean. Soap makes you smell good. Soap makes you beautiful and free from disease. And to prove it, only the most beautiful men and women are shown on TV and in the magazines.

The advertising departments of soap companies are not telling us all the facts about the harmful effects of soap. As the commercials say, soap kills germs. Germs are alive; germs are made up of one or more cells. What this means is that soap can kill living cells, including the living cells which compose your skin. When soap is placed in contact with your skin, the soap poisons the healthy, living skin cells, causing them to become diseased and die, just like germs.

Here I would like you to reconsider the true meaning of cleanness. *Webster's Dictionary* defines clean as something free from disease, free from matter that adulterates, contaminates or pollutes, free from dirt, filth, refuse or remains.

I am emphasizing the meaning of 'clean' because making yourself clean, inside and out, is the whole secret of tapping the fountain of youth.

The Skin Cell's Point of View

I have always heard that the skin is so tough. Skin *is* relatively waterproof. Skin is also remarkably germ-proof, but, of course, not completely so.

Skin is made up of individual living cells. Each cell knows exactly what it is supposed to do. It follows its DNA instructions as well as it can, given the external circumstances in which its owner has placed it.

Each cell is tiny—incredibly tiny. And it is also fragile. It is easily burned by exposure to sun or fire. It is always subject to being bumped and scraped by its owner's carelessness. It does not have long to live but must accomplish a great deal in a very short time.

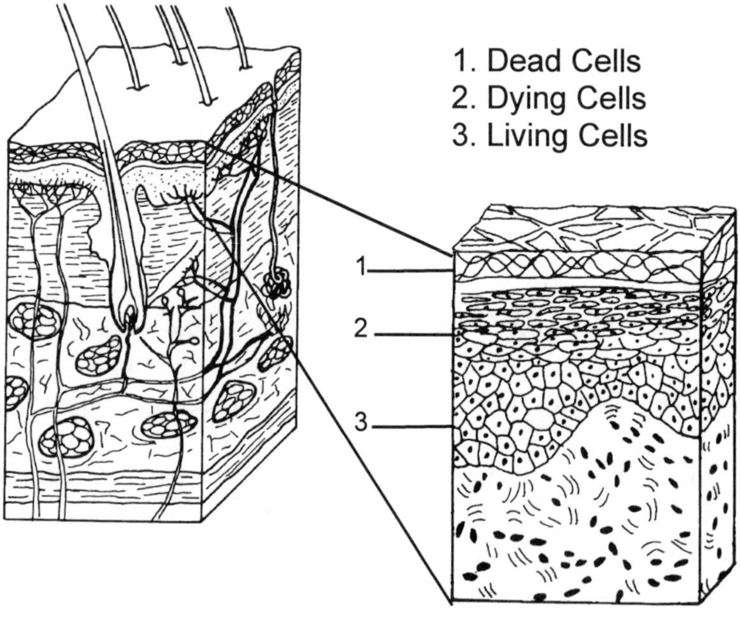

A minor scratch to the skin of a hand can kill hundreds of thousands of cells, and damage thousands of others. The cells which survive not only have to try to repair themselves, but are also still charged with their regular job of keeping the person to whom they belong healthy. So, if dirt and bacteria got in the scratch, it is, from the cell's point of view, an injury of catastrophic proportions.

Whatever happens to the person also happens to the person's cells. Skin cells are subject to extreme temperature changes, to air pollution, to changes in the light level from direct sunlight to total darkness.

Think what happens to the skin cells when the owner spends a day at the beach—in and out of the water all day, too much sun, the chafing of sand, the lotions and oils rubbed on. This is just too overwhelming for millions of cells. They simply die from one or more of the tortures caused by the relaxing day in the sun.

Let's look at soap and the most common agents we use to smell clean. Most soap is alkaline. If you have ever had even a little soap suds in your eye, you know how irritating the chemicals in soap can be. The chemicals in soaps can change the surface tension of the walls of the cells, causing cell membranes in the outer layer of skin to crack and break. The fluids within the cells dry up. The cells are literally evaporated to death. This becomes noticeable as dry skin.

Body powder is just talc, with some perfumes added. Talc is an abrasive, the same abrasive used in auto polishes. No matter how finely ground the powder is, it is still abrasive. Talcum powder feels so soothing and smooth when you put it on, but think of the cells whose fate is to live under the elastic bands of underwear, or anyplace where chafing occurs. Those poor cells must find talc particularly irritating.

Individual cells have no individual voice to complain, yet at the end of the day, many people find it feels so good to get out of their clothes.

Perfumes are a mixture of oils which are dissolved in alcohol. The oils may be natural or synthetic. Other chemicals are used to 'fix' the fragrance. Ambergris, a rubbery substance from the sperm whale, is the best known fixative. The alcohol in the perfume evaporates, leaving a thin layer of the other ingredients on the skin. Most of these eventually evaporate, too, but more slowly than the alcohol.

Cells are so small that being coated with face lotions and hand creams must seem to the cells like a major oil spill. We feel so sorry for an otter which has been caught in the black ooze of the Alaskan oil disaster. It's still alive, struggling to breathe. At the same time that we watch this emotional scene on TV, we may be doing nearly the same thing to our own living skin cells.

Your Skin's Best Friend

What makes your skin soft and healthy? The answer is your own natural body oil. By preventing the dehydration of individual skin cells, body oil prevents drying and cracking of the skin. *Your own body oil is your skin's best friend.* Body oil helps prevent the reproduction of germs and buffers the ill effects of outside hazards like poisonous chemicals.

If you rub your finger on the side of your nose and smell it, you will notice an unpleasant odor. This odor comes from fresh body oil (non-oxidized sebaceous material). Fresh oil loses this odor after a few minutes exposure to air because the oil oxidizes.

Washing with soap removes body oil and stimulates the glands to produce larger quantities of oil at a faster rate than normal. This over-production of oil induces more odor.

People who do not use soap do not have this problem. Since they do not stimulate oil production in this way, their natural oil production progresses at a rate slow enough for the oil to be sufficiently oxidized, thus producing less odor.

A swan can stay in the water for hours at a time because it applies its own oil to its feathers. This keeps its feathers healthy—and waterproof. If you caught a swan, washed the oil off its feathers with soap, then applied expensive cosmetics to the swan, would the swan be better off? Of course not. And yet, humans continually wash away their skin's best friend, body oil, with soap. Then they apply cosmetic creams, lotions, and oils, parts of which could be harmful, to replace this loss. Doesn't this seem rather foolish?

No replacement oil could possibly be as good for our skin as our body's own natural oil.

Please wake up! Save your skin! Stop washing with soap! Even if you 'wake up' now, and begin Skin Chunging, it will take a year to overcome the damage done to your skin by all the chemicals in the soap you have been using.

Skin Wrinkling and Skin Aging

If you compare healthy infant skin to wrinkly old skin, you will notice that the old person has a thicker dead skin layer, with spots of diseased skin here and there.

- If any of your friends over forty have no wrinkles, they probably do not use soap on their faces.

- If any of your friends are forty, and are so wrinkled they look as though they were sixty, chances are they have used soap on their faces more than once a day.

These two statements tell us a lot. Do not poison your skin with chemicals.

If you want to stop killing your skin, stop *unnecessarily* using soap. There are times, such as when you have gotten really dirty or greasy, when using soap is necessary—I do not mean to imply that soap should NEVER be used.

When you *do* use soap, extra rinsing with clean water is obviously a practical idea. It's important to get as much of the chemical residue off of your skin as you can. Remember, if you have washed with soap and have that nice, 'clean', perfumed smell of soap, it means you have not rinsed away the chemicals in the soap.

When you stop killing your skin, the layer of dead, dying, and diseased skin will eventually fall off. New, healthy cells constantly produced by the basal layer of your skin will replace this damaged layer, and after one year, your skin will be one year Chunger. After two years, your skin will be two years younger. After five years, your skin will be five years younger than today! For example, let's say you are now forty years old and at this point, you stop killing your skin. When you are forty-five, your skin will have better texture than it does now. In most cases, it should even be an improvement over your present complexion.

If you continue to do this, will your skin continue to look younger? No. From my observations, five years is the usual maximum. After that, if you continue Chunging, your skin continues to look young *for your age.*

Some Chemicals Go Through the Skin

You probably already know that there are medicines given in the form of skin patches, like ear patches for motion sickness, nitroglycerin patches for angina pain, and estrogen patches for post-menopausal women. And recently, there has been a great deal of advertising promoting patches to help people stop smoking.

The effectiveness of this form of dispensing medicine illustrates the fact that *skin cannot prevent* the penetration of certain chemicals into the internal body.

When soap comes in contact with your skin, it is probable that a portion, great or small, of the chemicals in the soap will get into your internal organs. I have not read nor heard of any research considering the possible effects of soap residue in the body, but I strongly believe that this should be studied.

Better Skin by Skin Chunging

Skin Chunging is based on these principles:

- Reducing the dead cell layer by slowly replacing it with living cells, rather than by removing dead cells from the surface of the skin by scrubbing.

- Preventing skin disease by avoiding contact with chemicals—including soap and cosmetics.

- Making skin cells healthier by promoting better blood and oxygen circulation.

No matter what age you are or the present condition of your skin, one year from the time you begin Skin Chunging, your skin will look and feel younger than you look today.

Skin Chunging

1. Make your skin cells clean by washing with water only. Don't contaminate your cells with unnatural chemicals. Do not wash with soap.

2. Do not cover up your skin with possibly dangerous cosmetics which may damage the cells. Avoid oils and deodorants which may block oxygen intake.

3. Rub your skin with your fingers and palms to increase circulation (not rubbing the skin's surface to create friction,

but rubbing in such a way that the layer of flesh under the skin is stimulated). This makes your subdermis healthier.

4. When you wash any part of your body, rub your skin only with your hands. This will ensure that you do not rub off your skin's protective barrier.

5. Do not scrub your skin with a washcloth, brush, or sponge. Do not try to remove the protective layer of dead skin. Wash by rubbing your skin with your hands only.

6. Gently pat yourself dry with a towel; don't rub your skin with a towel's rough, hard surface. The point is that dead skin should fall off naturally. Keep it as protection for the new and delicate skin cells underneath.

7. Wash as often as you like if you use only water. I recommend body washing once or twice a day in the summer and no more than once a day in the winter time. Most older people do not need to bathe every day. Do not stay in the water over 30 minutes because you may over-hydrate your skin cells. The liquid in the interior of skin cells has a greater concentration of electrolytes than water, allowing extra water to enter the skin cell, which makes the cells swell.

8. When you have been Skin Chunging a year, the layer of dead cells will be thinner. The new cells which have not been chemically damaged will have begun to replace the old cells which were damaged by the use of soap. I have never seen anyone who has been Skin Chunging for one year go back to using soap on their face and body. More than a thousand of my friends and patients are successfully Skin Chunging and feel really good about it.

When You Start Skin Chunging

The first three weeks after you stop using soap, you will probably feel very dirty and want to avoid close contact with others. This is partly psychological and partly physical. You *can* notice body odor at first.

The good news is that this is a temporary condition. You will have less and less odor as the dead skin is replaced with healthy skin. After three weeks, you won't feel as dirty. After three months, you will know that you are cleaner. At six months, any one who touches you is likely to comment that your skin texture is so soft it feels like velvet. People start commenting that you smell so good. In one year, you will be positive that Skin Chunging was a good move for you.

Don't Tell a Soul at First

I caution you that it may not be prudent to tell anybody about your new discovery. While you are just beginning Skin Chunging, people who have been told might assume that you were 'dirty'. They might make you self-conscious by trying to sniff you as they walk by, or tease you about your no-soap program. They might even avoid you. If this rejection were to persist, you would probably feel so uncomfortable that you would start using soap again, and as a consequence, start killing your skin again. So, my advice is: don't tell anyone when you start. It's nobody's business but yours. After you have proven to yourself the benefits of no-soap Skin Chunging, then feel free to discuss my ideas with your friends (and to recommend my book!).

Why Using a Wash Cloth is Bad for Your Skin

As you can see in the picture of the cross section of skin (page 32), the top layer (called the *stratum corneum)* is composed of a few layers of dead skin. These layers of dead skin serve the same purpose as bark on a tree; they act as a protective barrier for the delicate living cells in the layer below.

The only thing a wash cloth does is to rub off this protective coating.

If you rub off the protective layers of dead skin by abrading it with a wash cloth, you are exposing a tender, living cell layer called the *epidermis.* The epidermis, when exposed, will quickly die; in fact, it will die so quickly that the skin will probably still be slightly moist. You see this when a child scrapes a knee. This moist environment is an excellent culture medium for germ growth. You need the outer layers of dead and dying skin cells to protect the delicate live ones below.

Thus, by using a wash cloth, you are preparing yourself for disease. You would recognize this fact immediately if you could see the microscopic reality of your actions.

Shampoo is OK

Soap is good for cleaning dishes and clothes and things which are not living. Hair cells are already dead, and experiments eliminating the use of soap or detergent shampoos have left my patients' hair smelling dirty. What is true for the rest of the body, does not seem to apply to the scalp and the hair of the head. My conclusion is that it is all right to use shampoo.

I found the most difficult part in stopping the use of soap was to stop shampooing. It is so difficult that I usually tell my patients to simply use a mild shampoo and to rinse well. However, there are always a few brave patients who, after having such good results from the elimination of soap, attempt to stop using shampoo also. They are usually unsuccessful.

It took me three years to become comfortable not using soap or shampoo to wash my hair. For three years my hair carried a strong odor. However, after my third year, the odor began to dissipate. You *can* discontinue the use of shampoo, but I guarantee that it will be a long and difficult struggle. Most people prefer the 'clean' smell of freshly shampooed hair.

Skin Nutrition and Facials

Most people wish to appear young. They visit beauty salons to receive 'nutrition' through the skin.

But nutrition for the skin never comes from the outside; it only comes from the blood supply to the innermost layers of skin cells. Blood vessels in the dermis and subcutaneous tissue supply the nutrition and oxygen to those cells. The only good thing that comes from the outside is oxygen. Any other chemical only poisons the skin.

So, during a deep skin massage (in beauty salons), the only things that happen are that the protective layer *(stratum corneum)* is rubbed away, exposing the tender epidermis, and that toxic, cosmetic chemicals are rubbed into the epidermis in the name of nutrition. Because of this, the epidermal cells get sick, swell, then die.

As a result of the damage that facial massage does to the skin, the poor swollen cells cause the skin to temporarily appear less wrinkled and younger to the naked eye. These effects only last for a few hours or days, unfortunately. The 'younger look' only lasts until the body has had time to repair the damaged cells and replace the dead ones. This cellular damage to the skin is the reason why so many women develop facial skin problems like eczema and contact dermatitis a few days after an expensive trip to the beauty salon.

Why Antiperspirants Are Harmful

I hope that you will now understand that skin is a group of living cells; it is not 'dead' like leather, hair, or plastic. Living cells all have the same functions: they take nutrition, they digest, they work, and they excrete. In order for these functions to run smoothly, cells need oxygen.

If a person were choked and couldn't breath, he would die quickly. If someone has an intestinal blockage, and can't defecate, they might live a couple months in agony but would soon die. If one can't urinate due to one problem or another, the poisons in the body build up quickly and a painful death comes within a few weeks.

But this is exactly what you are doing to your skin when you use antiperspirant! You are coating living cells with a thick layer of chemicals (compared to the size of a tiny skin cell) in the hope that a product you buy will solve the odor problem. Instead, it is causing next week's B.O.

Sweating is like urination; both eliminate harmful waste products from the body. Therefore, sweating is one of the ways cells eliminate waste products. Skin exchanges oxygen with the air as well as with the blood. In this sense, use of deodorants causes cell choking. Blocking the elimination of waste causes the cells to die faster, which, in turn, accumulate as dead rotting cells, causing further body odor problems.

Only dying or diseased skin cells can create a foul body odor. Living healthy cells only produce beautiful aromas.

In people who have been Skin Chunging a year or longer, there are fewer and fewer dead cells in proportion to the healthy cells. Therefore, their perspiration does not have a strong offensive odor.

In summary, washing with water only, using no soap, and using no deodorant or antiperspirant is the correct solution to the body odor problem as well as the solution to keeping your skin young looking for your age.

It takes a few weeks from the time you first start Skin Chunging, but *it always works!*

Living Water

Everyone has to constantly refill his or her body with water.

Humans have lived 81 days without food but will die in five days without water. If a person loses 5% of his total water, he will start to hallucinate, become disoriented, and experience twitching muscles. If he loses 15% of his total water, his life is endangered.

I know how annoying the advice to drink water may seem. Many of my younger patients, those in their teens and early twenties, become annoyed when I tell them to "drink lots of water." Why? Because throughout their entire lives, they have heard nothing good about water. Newspapers and magazines have been constantly telling them that their water is contaminated and dirty. This negative publicity also causes their teachers and parents to worry about the quality of drinking water.

Simultaneously with this bad publicity about water, these people have been bombarded with glorious propaganda concerning soft drinks, coffee, tea, and beer. Ads imply that if you drink their product, you will be healthy and beautiful like the people in the photograph. Commercials make it seem like drinking the right beer will make you popular and happy. They almost always show a group of people having fun while drinking their brand of beer. The reality of a neighborhood bar is often quite different. Bars are full of lonely people. Laughter is few and far between. Even smiles are rare.

If they stop to think about it, most people realize that soft drinks are harmful. But apart from realizing that sugar and caffeine are not good, they do not really understand why soft drinks are so bad for their health.

The main difference between water and soda pop is that good drinking water has oxygen in it and soda has dissolved carbon dioxide gas under pressure, which forms the bubbles when you open the can or bottle.

A person breathes in oxygen and exhales carbon dioxide. Carbon dioxide, like urine and feces, is one of the waste products of the human body.

Drinking carbonated beverages adds large quantities of the very chemical the body is trying to get rid of.

If you take carbon dioxide into your system, your body tissue will absorb it. There just isn't room for both the carbon dioxide and the amount of oxygen each cell needs. The carbon dioxide pushes some of the oxygen out of the cell. The result is that the cell which is exposed to carbon dioxide goes through temporary hypoxia—lack of oxygen—which induces faulty metabolism. This eventually results in diseased organs.

Drinking soda keeps people from drinking water when they are thirsty. Soft drinks are harmful to your health because they do not cleanse your body's cells. Instead, chemicals in soda pop are accumulated within the cells as harmful waste products.

When I tell my patients that drinking water will help them stay healthy, some of them ask incredulously, "Do you mean Cincinnati water?" Yes, I mean regular, Cincinnati tap water. Then my patients tell me how contaminated city tap water is, and that it causes cancer.

If you go to any large city, most of the residents of that city will tell you that they have the dirtiest water in the U.S.A. Somehow, the media has convinced the majority of citizens that their water is too contaminated to drink.

I don't understand why these people believe that adding coffee, tea or other chemicals to their tap water will make the tap water any safer. The mixtures of chemicals in drinks *actually add contaminants* to the water.

Most people have all kinds of romantic pictures in their minds. They like to think that soft drinks are made from sparkling, splashing water which comes bubbling up from a pure spring somewhere far away in the mountains. They may imagine that there is a mystical fountain in a beautiful cave deep within Mother Earth where the bottlers go to make their delicious concoctions.

Some brewers and bottlers might use spring water carted in from some other location, but it's not likely—if it raised the cost of production much, they wouldn't spend the money. The vast majority of water used in making soft drinks comes either from the city water supply or from wells at the brewery, cannery, or bottling facility—wells which draw from the same aquifer as all the other wells in the community. City water comes from wells, springs, lakes, reservoirs, or from river water. If pollutants exist in the supply, it goes right into the bottled or canned product.

Whatever the source, *anything* that was in the water which was used in making soft drinks and beer, is still in it when you drink it. These drink manufacturers have added still more chemicals to make their products.

Rivers or reservoirs are sometimes contaminated with chemical spills, but a city's water is constantly tested by the engineers of the water department. Rural areas' water supplies are periodically checked by the counties. The counties are checked by the state. The Environmental Protection Agency also monitors the water all over the country to ensure the safety of the water supply. I don't think that the E.P.A. would allow people to drink anything as toxic as the media would lead us to believe.

Only water can clean waste products and toxic chemicals out of the body and out of the brain. If a person does not eliminate these waste products, it will cause disease and will alter his behavior in some way, sooner or later.

For example, since 1960, Americans' intake of soft drinks has increased and their intake of water has decreased. Also, due to air conditioning, Americans perspire less than they did in the past. During this time, the divorce rate has increased greatly, the quality of U.S. products has worsened, and the rate of drug abuse has increased. Of course, there are other reasons why these things have occurred. However, I believe the fact that Americans have greatly increased their intake of poisonous chemicals has played a major role in these phenomena.

Another example can be found in the fast-growing country of Korea. Until the 1980s, the Korean people were too poor to afford soft drinks. They were forced, financially, to drink water. Also, due to almost no air conditioning and a lack of cars, Koreans generally perspired heavily. During this time, their brains were very 'clean'—family bonds were tight, Korean industry was booming, and children were doing well in school. As Korea became richer, more problems developed. Now, in Korea, most people prefer soft drinks, many houses have air conditioning, and cars are becoming more easily accessible. The divorce rate is now climbing. Student protests are more violent than ever before, the crime rate is skyrocketing, and criminals are becoming more vicious. Workers do not wish to work, and employers do not wish to share. Again, the causes of these problems are complicated, but I believe that chemical intake and improper internal cleansing have been major factors.

A patient of mine who is an experienced grade school teacher told me that she used to spend her time teaching but now she feels stressed and angry as she has to spend most of her time keeping the students quiet and seated at their desks. She is depressed that she has so little time to teach them their lessons. I believe these bad actions on the part of the students are the result of the chemicals we parents introduce into their fragile brains by allowing children to drink soft drinks and to eat junk food loaded with artificial ingredients.

Living Water and Dead Water

Most Oriental health books recommend that you drink 'living water' but never explain exactly what they mean.

If you visit Seoul, Korea, you will see thousands of people awake in the early morning, 5:00 to 6:00 A.M., climbing nearby mountains for 30 to 60 minutes before going about their daily work. They go to the mountains to drink fountain water for better health. Most of them start this practice when they become sick. After doing this daily, many find that their illness begins to disappear and they become healthier. Because they feel good, they continue this morning routine.

To me this makes a lot of sense—walking daily for 30 to 60 minutes, breathing fresh mountain air, then drinking clean, uncontaminated, oxygenated fountain water. This is a good practice for anyone searching for better health.

Koreans call this uncontaminated fountain water 'living water,' its traditional name. The following are the definitions of living water and dead water:

- Living water is water which is compatible with life. Freshwater fish can live in it. It is the fresh rain water that sprinkles your garden. It is water which may contain some minerals but which certainly contains oxygen.

- Dead water is water which is not compatible with life. Distilled water and carbonated water are dead waters because fish die in them, even though those waters have no impurities. Plants, also, cannot live on dead water.

What causes the contradictory natures of essentially the same water is the amount of oxygen in the water. Water which contains the proper amount of oxygen is not harmful to fish and plants. Water which contains too little oxygen will kill those same fish and plants. When you put fish in water which has been boiled and cooled, the fish will die because boiling has removed the oxygen from the water

How to Oxygenate Water

If you don't have a bubbling fountain, you can easily cause oxygen to dissolve in water by stirring it in a blender, or by shaking it—fill a container about half full of water, put on a tight lid, and shake the container. This will properly saturate the water with oxygen to the right concentration.

One of the basic principles of homeopathy is that small quantities of medicines should be succussed; that is, medicines should be diluted and shaken. Homeopathic physicians observed, over the years, that this diluted and shaken medicine works better and they say this 'vitalizes' the drugs. I believe that the importance of shaking is to add beneficial oxygen to the mixture, as well as stirring up the contents.

I truly believe that before you drink water, you should shake it. If you do as I have described, your digestion as well as your general health will improve and you will be more resistant to diseases. You must not expect immediate results, but over the years it will benefit you. Many of the chemical processes which take place in the stomach and small intestine run more efficiently if there is enough oxygen present. Therefore, drinking living water also helps digestion.

Water Chunging

I recommend drinking six to ten eight-ounce cups of water per day for the average person, depending on their weight.

You must remember to balance the intake and output of water. Taking in too much water is as dangerous as dehydration. A person can become intoxicated by over-hydration. He will experience nausea, weakness, dizziness, trembling hands, cramping, and eventually would lose consciousness. You should not drink over twelve eight-ounce glasses (about 3000 cc) of water a day, except under special conditions.

One important rule of good health is "do not overdo," or "everything in moderation.". Even something known to be good for health can be dangerous if taken in too large quantities. Water, vital to life, can be harmful if consumed in excess.

Water and Aging

Doctors and researchers know that the main cause of aging is the accumulation of waste products in the body. The human body is composed of 100 trillion living cells. Each individual cell works and lives for you. To do this, each cell takes in nutrients, utilizes those nutrients, and discharges its waste products. Water then flushes the cells' waste products away.

The same is true of your whole body. You eat, digest, and wash away your excretions mainly with the help of water. When you wash your clothes, you fill your washer with water, not soft drinks, coffee, tea, or juice. Water is the only thing that can clean your clothes. The same mechanism applies to cleaning your body's cells. *Only proper amounts of water can clean your body's cells.*

I have encountered many people who take pride in saying, "I never sweat," or "I never drink water." I have observed that these people appear much older after the age of forty than people who sweat and drink water. By the age of fifty, many of them have become afflicted by arthritis or other 'incurable' diseases. Doctors can't completely cure these diseases because they don't yet know the causes.

When I meet people who are seventy-five and look twenty years younger, invariably I find that they sweat regularly and drink water.

In my opinion drinking plenty of water prevents the build-up of toxic waste in the body, thus expelling the cause of many diseases. Drinking lots of water also slows down the set of symptoms which we generally refer to as aging.

The cause of Alzheimer's disease is unknown at present. Researchers are aware that the nerve cells of people affected by this disease contain large amounts of unusual waste chemicals which eventually destroy the nerve cells. Eventually the number of nerve cells in the brain becomes drastically reduced, which causes the diminished abilities of thought and speech.

The brain lives in a liquid environment. I believe that, since drinking water minimizes waste accumulation in the brain, it can also help prevent Alzheimer's disease and other brain abnormalities. I wonder how people expect to clean their brain cells without enough water.

The environmental liquid with which the brain is surrounded is called spinal fluid. One of the signs of a fractured skull is some of this clear liquid leaking out of the ears. A spinal tap is also used to draw a small amount of this vital fluid in order to test for some brain diseases such as spinal meningitis. I only mention these things here to reinforce how important I believe it is to keep your brain clean by a constant intake of the most vital of thing of all—water.

Drinking enough water is an every-day-of-your-life thing. It is the essential ingredient for making all the Chunging exercises work for you. And like the other exercises I recommend, it is never too late to start drinking the proper amount of water; at any age, your body will definitely benefit.

Breathing

The first physical activity of human beings at birth is breathing. Breathing not only brings oxygen into your bodies, but it plays an almost equally important role in getting rid of harmful cellular waste.

If you don't breathe properly (inhale oxygen, exhale carbon dioxide), your cells will not be able to metabolize nutrition adequately, and will produce more toxic waste. Without proper breathing, physical exercise adds to the problem by producing more waste in the body than can be eliminated.

Over and over, I have seen that Western medicine is keenly aware of external sources of pollution, but neglects the internal source: waste produced by the cells themselves. If retained, the cells' own waste accumulates and begins to poison the body. This includes the waste product of breathing, carbon dioxide.

Proper breathing of fresh air is as important to health as drinking pure water. Consuming both clean air and clean water are ways of keeping the individual cells clean and functional. People who smoke are not able to properly exchange oxygen for carbon dioxide, and consequently, age faster and are more susceptible to diseases like cancer, heart attacks, blood clots, and strokes.

The Importance of Breath Chunging

There are two completely different types of breathing. They each require a different energy level and each serve quite a different purpose. You must understand these differences and *use the differences to your advantage.*

When a person becomes angry and excited, you may have noticed that you can actually see his chest heave as he gulps in air. This is called chest breathing and occurs when the walls of the chest actually expand and contract. It provides a faster way of exchanging oxygen and carbon dioxide.

During an emergency, chest breathing prepares you for faster action. A person will usually breathe through his or her mouth during chest breathing. It is high energy breathing, tiring if it is continued deliberately for a long period. Because it prepares the body for fight or flight, chest breathing is stressful.

Breathing that uses movement of the diaphragm rather than the chest wall is called diaphragmatic breathing. Also sometimes called abdominal breathing, it is visible by a bulging, outward motion of the abdomen when inhaling, and a sunken, inward motion when exhaling.

A young, healthy person uses his diaphragm to breathe most of the time. You usually cannot notice any movement of the

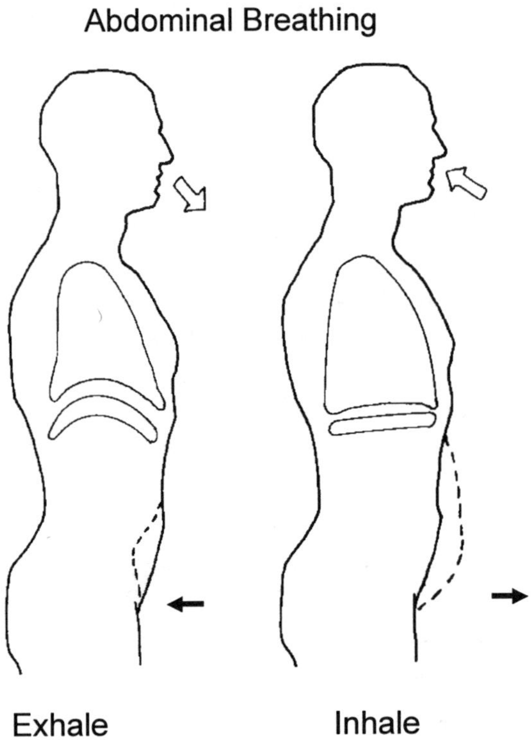

chest wall in people who breathe with their diaphragms; you can only see movement in the abdomen. When a person is relaxing or sleeping, he normally uses his diaphragm to breathe more than he uses his chest.

These two patterns of breathing have distinctly different physiological effects. When you breathe using your chest wall, you are exciting your sympathetic nervous system which raises blood pressure, makes your heart beat faster, and induces restlessness. These are good things in an emergency, but not for everyday life. When a person chest breathes in a non-emergency situation, he is adding stress to his life.

Chest Breathing is Unhealthy

Breathing with your chest is unhealthy because:

1. It consumes more energy than diaphragmatic breathing, making a person tired.

2. It stimulates the sympathetic nervous system, elevating blood pressure and inducing rapid pulse.

3. It allows less exchange of oxygen and carbon dioxide than in abdominal breathing. Although there is faster breathing, the breaths are shallow.

When you notice a healthy infant resting or sleeping, you will see that his abdominal movement is slow and rhythmic. When you watch an infant who is sick, you will notice that the infant's abdominal wall stands still; only the chest wall is expanding and contracting quickly.

An elderly person with lung or heart disease, or chronic illness, uses his chest wall to breathe more than he uses his diaphragm. Besides the discomfort and fear of not being able to breathe easily, chest breathing leaves the patient exhausted.

As a person gets older and weaker, there is a tendency to chest breathe rather than abdomen breathe. *Reversing this practice is one of the most important accomplishments of the Chunging exercises.*

Fortunately, you can reverse chest breathing by training. Breathing like a younger person will make you Chunger.

Breathing with your diaphragm will induce lower blood pressure, slower heart rate, and a calming of your emotions. Also, diaphragmatic breathing stimulates your intestines which helps digestion and circulation to your intestines.

I strongly recommend diaphragmatic breathing. Learn and practice abdominal breathing because it will give your body more oxygen and eliminate more carbon dioxide, remove stress, and calm your mind. These things keep you younger. Here is how it is done:

Breath Chunging

Breath Chunging is a cleansing activity. This breathing exercise can be done in any position, sitting, standing, or lying down, just so long as you are comfortable. If you have to stand in line at the grocery store, you could do a few Breath Chunging exercises while you are waiting. Since you have to breathe anyway, you might as well do it in such a way that it will do your lungs (and your whole body) the most good.

Breath Chunging is done as part of most of the other Chunging exercises. Proper breathing is crucial to all good exercise.

> Step 1. Exhale through your mouth slowly until there is no breath remaining; however, stop before you feel discomfort. When exhaling, open your mouth only the smallest amount you can. By doing this, you can keep the alveoli in your lungs inflated. Alveoli are the basic oxygen-carbon dioxide exchange units of the lungs. Alveoli look like tiny balloons. These balloon-like structures always have to be open to exchange air. By

breathing slowly through your mouth, you are creating resistance which causes the alveoli to stay inflated due to the back pressure.

Step 2. Then, close your mouth before you inhale so that you inhale through your nose. Allow your body to spontaneously, effortlessly, inhale through your nose. You will notice that your abdomen will bulge. Your chest must not expand during inhalation. In other words, don't breathe in deliberately.

Step 3. Hold your breath from one to thirty seconds. Before you feel uncomfortable, exhale slowly through your mouth, repeating the entire procedure.

Each time you breathe, you do not use all the oxygen you take into your lungs. Enough oxygen is left as you exhale, in fact, to support life in a person who is not breathing, by giving mouth-to-mouth resuscitation. The point of Breath Chunging is to get more of the oxygen you breathe into the cells where it will make metabolism more efficient.

Its important to inhale through your nose because the nasal cavity traps most of the contaminants in the air, such as pollen, dust, mites and allergens (things that cause allergies). The air reaching the alveoli must be clean. Always avoid dust, smoke, chemical fumes, even the odors from common household cleaners and heavily perfumed products of any kind. Many common products actually have dangerous volatile fumes. If a chemical is combustible, you should not breathe the fumes. Even breathing in a tiny amount of contaminants can easily damage the delicate surface of the alveoli, which will cause coughing and possibly future sensitivities.

The bronchus is the pipe-like passage through which air reaches the lungs. The bronchus also has the ability to trap airborne contaminants. Pollutants breathed in through the mouth overburden the bronchus, exposing it to disease and possibly allowing the development of bronchitis.

Inhaling slowly allows more time to trap dust and pollen so that cleaner air gets to the lungs. Your nose is equipped to trap this dust, protecting your lungs. The mouth does not have this ability. When you inhale with your mouth open, you are allowing harmful dust to enter your bronchus.

That is why slow and unintentional inhalation is so very important. Fast breathing does not allow enough time to trap all the contaminants when air passes through the nose, bronchus, and bronchioles, the smaller branches of the bronchus.

Several of my patients who suffered from headaches and nervousness claimed that these conditions became worse after deep breathing exercises which had been recommended by other physicians or friends.

I asked them to show me how they practiced deep breathing. All of them expanded their chests when inhaling, thus stressing their bodies through the sympathetic nervous system. Increased headaches and nervousness were the natural result of this sympathetic nervous system stimulation, brought on by chest breathing.

When you exhale properly, inhaling is spontaneous and restful, and your cells expel more waste. Due to the increased oxygen intake, more carbon dioxide can be expelled.

I hope I have convinced you about the importance of proper breathing.

From now on, when I say 'inhale' and 'exhale', I am referring to the Chunging Inhale and Chunging Exhale.

- **Chunging Exhale:** Open your mouth as little as possible. Exhale through your mouth as slowly as you can.

- **Chunging Inhale:** When you are finished exhaling, close your mouth. Let the air come through your nose slowly and spontaneously until your lungs feel comfortably full.

Proper Nutrition

As you know There are three sources of energy: carbohydrates (starch and sugar), protein, and fat. Which of these three can be metabolized with the least waste?

Carbohydrates

Carbohydrates are composed of only three elements: carbon, hydrogen, and oxygen. Carbohydrates are converted to glucose through enzyme action—and glucose is the main food of the body. When sugars and starches are utilized properly, they leave only carbon dioxide and water. Carbon dioxide is expelled from the body through the lungs. Water is expelled mainly through urine, perspiration and through breathing. In this way, carbohydrates leave no waste products; they are a very clean fuel source for body cells if there is enough oxygen.

Occasionally, the oxygen intake is insufficient, so that cellular oxidation of glucose cannot take place. Even under these adverse conditions, a small amount of energy can still be obtained, but glycolysis, because the conversion of glucose to pyruvic acid, does not require oxygen. Under anaerobic conditions (in which oxygen is not present), most of the pyruvic acid is converted into lactic acid, which remains in your cells until a surplus of oxygen is again available. This accumulation of lactic acid causes the feeling of tiredness.

Carbohydrates are one type of food that can be burned completely into carbon dioxide and water, both of which can easily exit the body and leave no waste in the cells.

Protein

Proteins are composed of nitrogen, carbon, hydrogen, and oxygen. You need twenty to thirty grams of complete protein per day. Usually, to be safe, sixty to seventy-five grams are recommended. If you consume more protein than you need a day, the excess protein will be converted to fat and stored in inconvenient places all over your body.

When protein is burned as energy, ammonia and urea are formed. These are undesirable end products, which, if allowed to collect in the body, may aggravate existing conditions or cause illness. Gout is the painful effect of a long term accumulation of these waste products. In uremia, a kidney disease, the kidneys have difficulty expelling the nitrogenous waste from the blood.

Even though they can produce toxic chemicals, proteins are extremely important because your body cannot synthesize all the amino acids which are necessary to life. You must ingest enough complete protein to supply all the essential amino acids. This is the meaning of the term complete protein: the twenty-one essential amino acids must all be present to be called complete. Meat, fish, poultry and beans are complete proteins. Vegetables contain some protein, but not necessarily all the amino acids essential to life. Corn, for instance, contains some protein, but it is lacking lysine, one of the essential acids. The deficiency disease pellagra is caused by a corn diet which lacks other protein.

Besides lysine, other common essential amino acids are tryptophan and tyrosine. Health food stores sell these and other individual essential amino acids as supplements. A few years ago, taking high amounts of tryptophan was a fad; a few people died from tryptophan overdoes before we learned that was not a good idea.

The same is true with the fabled protein diets. A number of people died from trying to live exclusively on these mixtures of powdered protein. These deaths did not occur in the distant history of medicine; this occurred within the past ten years.

Fat

Fat is a very cheap source of energy. However, unlike protein, only a small amount of fat intake is essential because a normal body can produce almost all the types of fatty acids that it needs.

When the body utilizes fat for energy, ketones and other toxic wastes are created. In persons suffering a diabetic crisis or on a 'starvation' diet, ketones may be detected on their breath as a fruity odor.

It is known that an excess of fat makes it difficult for many organs to function properly. For example, in diabetes, fat interferes with the passage of sugar into the body cells, causing the sugar to remain in the blood rather than being utilized in the cells. This is one of the factors in diabetes which causes the high blood sugar level. Other important forms of fat, cholesterol and triglycerides, cause heart disease by blocking arteries.

In Leviticus 7:23, the Lord said to Moses, "Say to the Israelites: Do not eat the fat of the cattle, sheep, or goats."

Why has it taken us so long to act on this good advice?

Vitamins and Minerals

In order to utilize nutrients, your body cells need oxygen and enzymes. If there is a lack of oxygen, metabolism becomes extremely inefficient and produces more toxic waste. If there are no enzymes, metabolism cannot even take place. Enzymes are organic chemicals produced in your body, which cause other chemical reactions to take place or to take place more efficiently. In order to protect yourself from this type of poisoning (waste build-up caused by lack of enzymes), you must take in a proper amount of vitamins and minerals, as they are the building blocks of the enzymes you continuously produce and use.

The main minerals which are necessary are calcium, potassium, phosphorus, sodium, and iodine. Calcium and phosphorus are used to make bone and cartilage. Calcium in the blood is used by the muscles.

These minerals are used by the body and then are excreted. So, you constantly need a new supply.

Ingesting just the right amount of these minerals—neither too much nor too little—is essential to your health. Each of these minerals is a poison if taken in too large a dose. Therefore, it is important to take supplementary vitamins and minerals under the supervision of your physician.

Eating Habits of Children

The eating and water-drinking habits of children depend upon parents. If adults feed children salty foods and chemically contaminated drinks, they will learn to enjoy these tastes and may later abuse them. Perhaps you never thought of soft drinks and salt as chemicals—but they are.

Craving salt is largely a matter of habit. Children who are used to it might miss salt when they first cut back, but humans are adaptable and after a short time on a lowered salt intake, food tastes fine without the extra salt.

The main objectional ingredients in pop are sugar, artificial coloring and flavoring, preservatives, and caffeine. Besides the long-term damage to teeth, sugar and possibly some of these other ingredients are known to cause many children to become temporarily hyperactive.

Read the labels! Artificial sweetener and artificial color and artificial flavor are all just that—artificial. Adult humans don't need all these unnecessary chemicals and certainly children don't. Their bodies may not have the ability to cleanse all the artificial products out of their cells. Don't risk your child's future by allowing him to become addicted to pop and junk food.

Strenuous exercise causes an increase in the production of cellular waste. Unless children drink water, this increased amount of cellular waste cannot be properly washed away. Drinking water is a good habit for children to develop; if they are always given sweet drinks when they are thirsty, they will never learn how delicious water really is.

Conclusions on Nutrition

The cleanest energy source is carbohydrate. Both protein and fat produce more waste and more toxic waste.

Marathon runners consume large amounts of carbohydrates because carbohydrates leave almost no waste in the body. Marathon runners seem to be all muscle, no fat. Yet at the end of a long race, they are bent over with pain—pain caused by the build-up of waste products in their bodies. They were burning fuel at a rate much faster than the rate at which they could get rid of the toxic waste their bodies were creating. No waste, no tiredness.

A person who is Chunging will eat more vegetables, fruits and cereals. He will avoid fat intake as much as possible. He will eat less meat than he used to consume. And of course, he will drink lots of water. Knowing what is good for you is one thing, but only you can choose to do what is right for your own body. You are in charge of your own life.

Chemical Sensitivity

Toxic chemicals are any chemicals which we don't need, or too much of a chemical which we do need. Do not think of toxicity only in terms of exotic poisons; almost anything can be toxic if ingested in large enough quantities—and even a microscopic amount may be a large enough dose to harm you.

Toxic chemicals are introduced to the body from both external and internal sources. Externally, toxic chemicals are either eaten, drunk, inhaled, or absorbed through the skin or mucous membranes of the mouth, nose, vagina, or rectum.

The internal source of toxic chemicals is more complicated. Internally, toxic chemicals come either from overproduction of normal, needed chemicals which are manufactured in various parts of the body, or from metabolizing non-toxic food chemicals as waste.

Your body is composed of trillions of living cells. Each individual cell takes in nutrients, utilizes the nutrients, and discharges its waste. If this waste is not cleaned away with water, the waste collects in different organs, and depending on the nature, location and quantity of the chemical waste, different illnesses show up in the person.

These symptoms of illness may be physical, such as pain, gas, diarrhea, or headaches. They might appear as psychological abnormalities, such as extreme anger, depression, or anxiety. Some symptoms could be mental and show up as confusion or forgetfulness.

Insulin is a good example of an internal toxic chemical which drastically affects the body. Insulin is needed to control the use of sugars in the body. The body manufactures this chemical in the pancreas. If the body produces too much insulin, severe hypoglycemia (low blood sugar) might result. If it produces too little, the results are equally devastating. This condition, the production of too little insulin, is called diabetes. One of the symptoms of diabetes is a craving for water—people with diabetes drink lots and lots of water. It is the body's own way of trying to correct the chemical imbalance by diluting the high concentration of sugar in the blood.

The margin for the body's requirement of other essential chemicals is also remarkably small. Potassium is an example of an external source of a toxic chemical. The element potassium is essential for life, but only a tiny amount is required. Again, either slightly too little or a small amount too much results in a wide variety of maladies. Either too much or too little could cause death. Potassium is a strong poison—*and yet we have to have some to live.* The same thing is true of iodine; everyone knows iodine is a deadly poison, yet we have to have a little. Normally we get enough potassium from foods such as bananas and orange juice, and enough iodine from seafood and iodized salt.

Sensitivities

Everyone has different sensitivities towards chemicals. Most people now recognize that smoking is bad for us and that excessive use of alcohol leads to health problems. We are exposed to many chemicals every day in household cleaners, in lawn and garden chemicals, pesticides, and in chemical additives to food and drink. When there is a problem, it is difficult to figure out the real cause.

The reason why one person is more sensitive to a particular chemical mixture than another person may have to do with the other chemicals to which that person has been exposed. This exposure may be accidental, such as spilling a pesticide on the skin, or deliberate, like drinking orange soda pop.

There are several factors in chemical sensitivity: how the chemical was introduced into the body (by ingestion, inhalation, or skin contact), how much of the chemical was present, and whether a dangerous dose was introduced all at once or over a period of time.

The harmful chemicals which are most commonly introduced to the body over a long period of time are those found in food and beverages. Consider what a coffee drinker puts in his system over his lifetime.

The point I want to make here is that although you might have a higher tolerance to chemicals than other people, prolonged use of these chemicals will still harm you. Absolutely no one is completely invulnerable to the accumulation of synthetic and harmful chemicals in the body.

Coffee and Tea

It is common knowledge that caffeine is not only addictive but is a poison. Too much will kill you. However, even a little caffeine will have the following effects:

1. It burdens the heart by increasing the heart rate and blood pressure.

2. It increases the secretion of stomach acids which cause stomach ulcers.

3. It augments emotional distress and insomnia.

4. It is a probable cause of many diseases like fibrocystic disease of the breasts (lumpy breasts).

When a person develops the above-mentioned ailments, the first thing the doctor advises is to stop drinking coffee. People dismiss this advice, saying to themselves "I only drink a couple of cups," or "a little coffee can't hurt me."

Caffeine causes irregular heart beat, commonly called 'heart palpitations'. If a person with irregular heart rhythm drank 20 cups of coffee in one hour, he might die. Of course, you are not likely to do that. But many people drink 10 to 12 cups a day, year after year, even after they have signs that the caffeine is affecting their heart.

Again, the healthy person says, "it can't hurt me." With this attitude, the person drinks his four or five cups of coffee every day. It may not kill him, but it certainly does its damage.

Soft Drinks

When a person develops bladder or kidney trouble, his doctor will tell him to stop drinking soft drinks and to drink only water. If a healthy person drank too much soda pop in one day, it is very probable that the person would find blood in his urine the next day. This is a very frightening experience for anyone.

The body has a well-balanced electrolyte system. Electrolytes are liquids or solids that conduct electricity by a flow of ions. When you drink soft drinks, you are introducing foreign electrolytes into your body system, upsetting the natural chemical balance. In order to compensate for this, your kidneys start working overtime. In passing these unnatural, poisonous electrolytes, your kidneys become damaged. Your whole body suffers from this invasion of unnatural chemicals.

Many people think that caffeine-free, diet soft drinks are safer than regular soda pop. I'm afraid, however, that the synthetic chemicals in these diet drinks (such as sweeteners, coloring, preservatives and so on), once ingested, cannot be completely expelled from the body after the body cells absorb these chemicals. To do no damage, these chemicals should enter and leave the body without leaving behind any residue.

Researchers have continuously been unable to account for 100% of the excretion of any chemical ingested which cannot be metabolized. Much of these chemicals are discharged from the body—but not every microscopic bit. I believe, therefore, that the body retains a small fraction of every synthetic chemical ingested, at least for a time, and that these chemicals may accumulate to interfere with cellular function. Again, look at it from the cell's point of view. It would take a very small amount indeed of a synthetic chemical to drastically change organized cellular function. How many cells could you afford to have not working properly—and still feel your very best?

Environmentalists say that the earth is becoming a garbage can because man-made substances such as plastics cannot be broken down and recycled by nature.

It is my belief that some synthetic chemicals found in soft drinks, food substitutes, and drugs may act almost like plastics in the environment. The body tries to eliminate plastic-like chemicals, but they are not biodegradeable, so they build up as waste.

Likewise, synthetic chemicals can only build up as waste in your system. Although the effects of this waste may not be immediate, as the waste accumulates permanent damage may occur in the future. This is one of the reasons I strongly advise you to use medicine only when absolutely necessary.

Perspiration

For most Americans, especially for women, sweating represents an unpleasant bodily experience. It makes their body odor stronger, makes their skin sticky, and ruins their facial make-up.

Western doctors say the main function of sweating is to cool the body by evaporating water from the skin's surface when body temperature becomes elevated by physical exercise and a hot environment. The other minor functions of sweating are considered insignificant. They believe sweat is unnecessary if body temperature is normal.

Due to these concepts regarding perspiration, there are many sophisticated, well-educated women who are proud of themselves for the fact that they 'never sweat', which means to them that their body doesn't smell, their skin is dry and soft, and they are an emotionally calm and cool person. Staying calm does cause less sweating and produces sweat that is milder in odor. To ensure that they 'never sweat' most American women use anti-perspirant to block the secretion and excretion of sweat.

However, to me, and to most Oriental physicians, sweat is perceived as always pleasant and beneficial, because it represents good health and cure of disease. Sweating is one of the major prescriptions of Oriental medicine. They say "make yourself have a good sweat, and your illness will disappear."

During my childhood in Seoul, Korea, whenever I caught a cold or flu and suffered from fever and body aches, my grandmother wrapped me with warm blankets until I had a good sweat. This made my fever come down by cooling evaporation and made my body aches disappear. I always thought that sweating eliminated the poison or the cause of the fever from my body.

In Western medicine, when a person has a high fever, body aches, and other symptoms of the flu, the doctor gives him medicine like aspirin, acetominophen, or ibuprofen. This treatment keeps the fever down and eliminates body aches. Since the patient then has no symptoms of the disease, he can continue with his normal activities.

I feel that the Western treatment of the flu (take an aspirin and go back to work) only makes the person more run down. By eliminating the symptoms but not the cause, the person feels good enough to act as though the disease were not present. This only makes the person more tired, and consequently, more sick. A young person whose body is still relatively strong can use the Western method of flu treatment with no difficulty. However, an older person receiving the same treatment can have serious complications.

There are two types of sweat glands, eccrine and apocrine. Each has different functions and expels different chemicals.

Eccrine or Passive Perspiration

Passive perspiration is induced by environmental hot temperatures such as a sauna or hot tub. This is called eccrine sweating.

Eccrine sweating can be beneficial to the treatment of disease, but only if you are exposed to the high temperatures for a short time. If you perspire in the high temperatures for more than five minutes, you may produce an imbalance in your electrolytes, a chemical imbalance which could lead to a heat stroke.

Eccrine sweat glands are located all over the human body. They regulate temperature through evaporation. Eccrine sweat is made of water and an electrolyte mixture containing salt, potassium, bicarbonate, and inorganic compounds such as lactate, urea, and ammonia.

Secretion of water not only controls body temperature, but also eliminates large quantities of salt. Therefore, eccrine sweating tends to act as an anti-hypertensive agent which helps the body prevent and cure high blood pressure.

The lactate in sweat is a metabolic end product of carbohydrate and fat. If retained, lactate acts as a poison, so it is important to get the lactate out of your body. Perspiring flushes the excess lactate out of your system.

Urea and ammonia in sweat are the metabolic end products of the utilization of protein. If retained, these chemicals cause the diseases commonly called uremia and gout which cause severe pain, seizures, and coma.

Any poisonous chemical, germ, or virus, once introduced into the human body, must somehow be expelled from the system to prevent and cure illness. Sweat glands are one of the body's major exits for these disease-causing agents.

Some chemicals mainly get out of the system through the sweat glands. For example, several hours after a single oral dose of fungicidal medicine is administered, a high concentration of the drug is observed in the skin. This drug is actually secreted into the sweat.

I firmly believe that in any viral disease which induces fever and skin rash, the sweat glands provide an exit for the virus. For instance, when the measles or chicken pox virus gets into the patient's blood, the body's fight against the invader makes the patient feel sick and get feverish. The fever induces sweating, which gets the virus out of the body through the sweat. If the viral population is too high for the skin cells to handle, damage to the skin cells can subsequently produce skin rash and eruptions. Doctors find the highest viral concentration under skin eruptions, which are very infectious. When the eruption is healed, the measles or chicken pox virus has departed from the patient's body and the patient is cured.

One of medicine's big mysteries is why any fever-producing drugs can cure the illness manifested by a fever. This medical fact has been confirmed by both Western homeopathy and the Eastern medical profession for many centuries, but neither group has explained why it is true.

I propose a simple explanation based on the physiology of sweating. Any type of fever induces body sweating, and the sweating then expels the causative factor of the febrile illness.

Fever is a natural body defense which pushes the virus to the skin level from deep inside the body. Sweating then dumps enough of the viruses outside the body that the body's own defenses can handle the rest. When the cause does not exist anymore, the disease is cured. But this sweat does not carry a high enough concentration of the virus to be infectious like the skin eruption.

Even human immuno-virus (HIV) may go out of the body through sweating. This may explain why athletic people who are affected by HIV stay healthier and live longer. They reduce the total number of virus in the body by sweating more frequently than those who have a more sedentary life style

I believe that many diseases with an unknown cause in which researchers have found unidentified viruses present in the diseased person (such as chronic fatigue syndrome, rheumatoid arthritis, and many cancers), are benefited by sweating. It is my observation that the person who sweats regularly is less likely to be involved with this kind of illness.

There are several cases from around the world in which AIDS patients were spontaneously cured without apparent reason. Logically, this cure only can happen when all of the HIV disappears from the patient's body. Somehow, nature found an exit for the HIV or destroyed it in these patients.

Doctors are researching how a virus enters the body, what it does inside of the body, and how a virus harms a human. However, I do not think they are paying proper attention to how the virus *gets out of* the patient. I hope this new concept of mine stimulates researchers. It may be much easier on the body to clean viruses out of the patient, rather than to kill viruses inside the human body with drugs, many of which have such drastic side effects.

I have noticed that many of my patients with depression and anxiety found that they were helped by drinking more water and sweating by following exercises which I recommended. These changes in their lifestyle worked because they diluted and removed depression-causing chemicals.

I believe that much more research should be done to correlate abnormal chemicals in perspiration with various types of depression. Researchers have already found an unusual chemical, hexonoic acid, in the sweat of patients with schizophrenia. Schizophrenia is an extreme disease, of course. But mild depression is so common, it deserves much more attention than it currently gets.

Another benefit of sweating is healthier skin. Sweat lactate and urea may be instrumental in the moisturization of the skin by promoting hydration of the *stratum corneum*, and by enhancing epidermal shedding through its keratolytic effect, which prevents a skin disease called hyperkeratosis.

Apocrine or Active Perspiration

Active perspiring refers to perspiration due to exercise. This type of perspiration utilizes both types of sweat glands, eccrine and apocrine. It works better than passive sweating in preventing disease. Sweating from active work or sports is very healthy and almost never causes the problems that can arise from passive perspiration alone.

The apocrine sweat gland, usually associated with hair follicles, continuously secretes a fatty sweat and is controlled by the adrenergic nerves. Emotional stress expels the fatty sweat on the skin. The chemicals in this type of sweat have a specific odor which, in animals, works to attract the opposite sex.

In humans, the apocrine glands are concentrated under the arms and in the genital region. In humans, apocrine perspiration also acts as an aphrodisiac.

This fatty sweat, however, can be contaminated by bacteria and disease. Bacteria may break down the fatty secretion into an unpleasantly pungent fatty acid. It is *this* sweaty odor that has sold millions of dollars worth of chemical 'cover-ups'. *This* bad sweaty odor, as well as the effects of the deodorants which are applied to the problem, totally overwhelms and hides the delicate allure of the aphrodisiac effect.

One of my friends, a Caucasian physician, told me of his experience. One Sunday morning, when he was awaking, he noted a very good, unusual aroma around him. He looked for the origin and found it was his underarm. He had been doing my Skin Chunging, no soap and no anti-perspirant, for over one year.

Please let your sweat glands work for you. Do not block the normal flow of sweat with anti-perspirants. Blocking the flow of nature produces only one thing: disease. Skin Chunging will minimize skin bacteria and therefore there will be no skin disease. Remember, only diseased skin and abundant bacteria produce foul body odor. Healthy skin has a good smell, a clean odor which does not come from soap.

Sweat Chunging

Some of the best ways to induce active sweating, if you are under forty, are racquetball, jogging, and bicycling. Over the age of forty, try riding an exercise bike until you sweat. Even better, you should do deep knee bends (described in the chapter on "Adult Diabetes") and sit-ups (described in "Spine Chunging"). You must remember to drink sufficient water before and after passive sweating, and after active sweating, not before. I mean *water*, not tea or soda. The accelerated metabolism during physical exercise and the heated body produce large amounts of metabolic end products which require water to be flushed out, and the body needs to be refilled with fresh clean water to replace the dirty water which was lost by sweating.

There are many women who claim “I cannot sweat, even if I try." I found that most of them do not drink sufficient amounts of water. Without water you can’t sweat.

There are a few athletes who sweat regularly who do not drink water, but only drink soda. They may easily develop disease and violent emotion since they are not properly washing away the end products of metabolism, which can induce disease as well as abnormal emotion.

However, you must not over-sweat because it could induce an imbalance of body electrolytes that can prove harmful. That is the reason athletes drink mineral-replacing fluids during hard workouts. There is a greater need for fluids when exercising in hot weather, so drink plenty of cold water.

Swollen Brain Syndrome

What causes the brain to swell? I believe that there are four factors which contribute to brain swelling:

1. Salt.

2. Carbonated beverages and other junk food.

3. Lack of water intake.

4. Lack of exercise (no perspiration).

Regardless of sex, age, education, or wealth, any person whose lifestyle includes these factors in excess, will exhibit abnormalities in behavior similar to those found in women suffering from PMS.

Good examples of the swollen brain syndrome can be seen at the high school level. Generally, there are three groups of students in most high schools. The 'good' group tend to be cooperative with their peers and teachers, study for their classes, and tend to veer away from illegal actions.

Students in the 'bad' group do not share these tendencies; they disrupt the classroom by irritating other students and pestering the teacher. They have no desire to study or learn, and they rebel against any authority for no apparent reason. They often use, to some extent, illegal drugs such as alcohol and marijuana. They believe their behavior is 'cool'.

The third and largest group include students who fall somewhere between these two extremes.

People from both extreme groups may have the same environmental, social, and economic backgrounds. But if you study their diet and exercise patterns, you will see an enormous difference between the two groups.

> 'Good' Group—Children who drink proper quantities of water, exercise daily, and consume very few soft drinks and little salty food find it easier to be responsible, compassionate, and logical.
>
> 'Bad' Group—Children who drink very little water, get little exercise, who drink only soft drinks, and who eat very salty foods, find themselves engaged in rebellious and illegal acts. These children suffer from swollen brains.

By abuse of harmful chemicals, I do not mean only addictive drugs. I mean the overuse of the unnatural chemicals which are routinely added to our food and drink, such as preservatives, artificial additives and synthetic flavors, sweeteners, and coloring agents—read almost any label on any grocery store shelf. The list of things manufacturers add, especially to junk food, is enormous.

A similar grouping can be found in marriages. There are generally two types of marriages:

> Happy marriages—Each partner loves the other and they plan together to accomplish things in the future.
>
> Unhappy marriages—They don't think they love each other. They never think about their future together. They think only of their individual futures, and they often consider divorce.

Obviously, there are many other reasons for divorce; however, the effects of abnormal chemicals on the brain would make any marriage difficult. People with swollen brains simply cannot handle loving relationships.

Altered Brain Chemistry

What begins as a purely chemical condition causes a physical problem which, in turn, results in psychological problems.

An excess of salt and other abnormal chemicals, which occasionally causes hands and ankles to swell, makes one feel fat and bloated, maybe headachy. If the swelling continues, it can cause actual pain to the point that the person can't even walk. When a person takes in an excess of salt and other abnormal chemicals, it *also* alters the chemical balance in the brain.

In order to dilute and flush out these chemicals, the body adds extra fluid to the brain. This extra fluid causes the brain to swell, and press against the skull. In addition to the chemical imbalance, actual physical pressure builds up in the brain.

In the early stages of a swollen brain, the person feels irritated. Because the brain is encased in its bony cage it cannot expand outwardly as the ankles do. If the condition continues, the person can progress from irritation to unreasonable fury.

Altered brain chemistry and swollen brains are why so many marriages in the unhappy group have such serious problems. Since people in one family tend to have somewhat similar eating habits, a husband and wife with swollen brains will fight continuously and be unhappy with their lives. Their children will probably have swollen brains from sharing their parents' diet, and they will have the added handicap of growing up in an unhappy household. What chance do these children have at a good life themselves?

Behavior and emotion are largely dependent on brain chemistry. Everyone knows that both alcohol and marijuana can *drastically* alter behavior. But little thought is given to what preservatives in hot dogs or soda pop might do to the brain. Brain chemistry is so incredibly complicated that science is just beginning to understand the subtle changes which drastically affect personality. Chemical imbalance and swollen brains cause emotional swings and mood changes. If you are depressed, there are chemicals in your brain causing it. If you are angry, chemicals in your brain are causing anger.

Most doctors attempt to eliminate distressing emotions by counteracting them with other chemicals such as mood elevators and tranquilizers.

Physicians *should* begin their treatment of patients by first eliminating the abnormal chemical agents from the patient's system, as opposed to merely counteracting them with drugs.

PMS

As a gynecologist, I consult daily with women suffering from mild to severe cases of Pre-Menstrual Syndrome (PMS).

There are numerous theories at present explaining PMS, but to me, none are totally convincing. There are also many treatments for PMS, such as tranquilizers, mood elevators, hormones, and diuretics. Although these treatments seem to work, they are only temporarily solutions. Afterwards, the symptoms always return in full force. Obviously, what is needed is a method to entirely eliminate the problem.

So, I began to investigate PMS myself. First, I asked my patients to describe their symptoms to me. Their symptoms typically included depression, crying, anger, and other emotional outbursts which occurred without apparent cause and which they could not control.

During PMS, my patients felt like they were different people. In describing themselves and their actions during PMS, they often said they felt like a 'bitch' or that they acted 'bitchy,' always regretting the episodes later. When I analyzed these responses in detail, I found five distinct groups of symptoms. Some, fortunately, may appear only in the most severe cases of PMS.

Some women have one or any combination of these symptoms:

- After ovulation, a woman begins to gain water weight, frequently five to ten pounds, which is expressed as bloating of the lower abdomen and enlargement and tenderness of the breasts.

- Women suffering from PMS often have an irrational desire to be alone. If a friend wants to talk or play tennis, a woman suffering from PMS will usually brush her off or ignore her.

- Women suffering from severe PMS cannot handle loving or close working relationships.

- A women suffering from severe PMS can only think in negative, destructive terms. She may break things, slam doors, or in other ways let everyone know she is angry. Or she may become quiet and not speak to her spouse. When a woman suffering from severe PMS has a fight with her husband, the woman often starts entertaining thoughts of divorce, instead of thinking about resolving their conflict

- When the PMS sufferer has trouble at work, she can only think negatively, and comes up with some sort of revenge against some slight or imagined wrong. She may 'tell people off', or even, in a rage, quit her job.

- Although they can still distinguish between right and wrong, women suffering from severe PMS tend to do 'wrong' things. For instance, they might:

    1. Abuse their children.

    2. Use foul language towards family and friends.

    3. Be caught shoplifting.

    4. Behave anti-socially in some other way.

Although these women regret their actions immediately, they explain that they simply could not stop themselves from doing these wrong acts.

PMS: Relationships with Children

If woman's own child came to her wanting to play or asking for a cookie, the woman with severe PMS would probably become very angry and scold the child about one thing or another. There is *always something wrong* with any person or any situation in the mind of a woman in this condition. Behavior of the child which would be ignored or gently corrected the rest of the month is jumped upon by the PMS sufferer. "Making a mountain out of a molehill" is the common reaction to anything the poor child does or says.

If the child continued to bother the woman, she might slap the child or jerk the child violently by the arm. A smart child soon learns to disappear after one of these unwarranted attacks, and goes outdoors or to his room to sulk or cry.

Surprisingly enough, if it were a neighbor's child who came to the woman with the same request, the woman would fulfill the child's request with no expression of anger.

This strange phenomena of reacting wrongly to the people closest to them and yet being kind to strangers is one of the worst effects of severe PMS.

PMS: Relationships with Husbands

Many women have this experience during PMS: when the husband first comes home and the woman hears the door open, the woman, for no apparent reason, becomes slightly irritated. As she hears her husband approaching, her anger mounts. When the husband finally greets the woman, the woman stares coldly at her husband for a moment then ignores him. If her husband asks what is wrong, the woman is liable to go into hysterics and begin to cry or vent her increasing anger in one way or another.

During severe PMS, it is nearly impossible for a husband and wife to hold a reasonable conversation without the wife suddenly bursting into fits of either crying or screaming without any reasonable cause.

However, if this same woman were to meet a complete stranger at a party, she could very easily hold a pleasant conversation with him.

The woman then begins to wonder why she can't discuss anything with her husband, and yet, she can easily communicate with a stranger. She begins to blame her husband for his inability to communicate. Soon she even begins to doubt his love for her, and her love for him. A woman in this state of mind is very much at risk; many casual, dangerous affairs start during PMS.

Unhappy thoughts doubting her husband's love fade as the PMS days pass. The woman really loves her child and husband, which, for some strange reason, is why she can't tolerate them.

The woman has no such connection with the stranger, which is why she can be nice to him. Women suffering with PMS often exhibit this love/hate relationship; they simply cannot tolerate loving relationships

Reversal of Behavior

After menstruation, women who suffer from PMS experience a complete reversal of behavior:

1. The bloating subsides. The breast tenderness totally disappears.

2. Women, after menstruation, become energetic and sociable.

3. Women who suffer from severe PMS, after menstruation, no longer rebel against people they love. They want to show their affection towards the very people to whom they were unkind during their affliction with PMS. They no longer feel alienated from friends and family or seek comfort from strangers.

4. They think positively and can work productively.

5. After menstruation, women who suffer from severe PMS, again have control over their actions. If they know what is right, they will *do* what is right.

A woman suffering from PMS, especially severe PMS, experiences two distinct personalities. Her family, friends, and co-workers have to cope with these cyclical changes in her behavior. One part of the month she is her normal, kind self. But a few days every month, she is like someone they don't know. She flies off the handle at trivial incidents, is unkind in the way in which she says things, she neglects her friends--perhaps it is not surprising that she describes herself as a 'bitch'.

She hates being this way. She takes over-the-counter medicines, and she *tries* not to get angry, but flies into fits of anger anyway. She seeks medical attention, and gets prescriptions that may help for that particular month, but the medicine does not eliminate the recurrence of PMS again the next month.

The Physiology of Menstruation

The only way to understand the radical, periodic shifts in personality which occur in women suffering from PMS is to study the physiology behind menstruation.

After ovulation (until menstruation), a woman has a higher amount of estrogen and progesterone in her body. These increased levels of hormones induce many physiological changes, including a retention of salt and water. Retaining salt and water inhibits the normal flushing of cellular waste from the body. This is simple cause and effect; retention of water and cellular waste causes the weight gain, bloating, and the swollen and tender breasts.

Water retention also occurs in the brain, causing the brain to swell. Anyone whose brain is swollen with cellular waste will have the same behavior and personality change as do women suffering from PMS, regardless of age or sex. For example, a person who just underwent brain surgery would display characteristics of personality change normally found in women suffering from PMS because, due to the manipulation of his brain tissue, that person's brain would be swollen.

The retention of cellular waste also explains why women suffering from PMS feel better after exercise or crying. Women do cry about four times more often than men. Basal tears—tears of lubrication—are quite different chemically from reflex tears, which are tears of emotion. Reflex tears (and perspiration) are basically 'salt water'. The release of this salt water from their bodies through crying or sweating during exercise helps to reduce the amount of cellular waste, and as a result, makes the woman feel much better.

This physiological change each month is nothing new. Primitive women probably also had mood swings at that time of the month. What *is* new, and what undoubtedly greatly effects the drastic swings of mood and personality which we now see in extreme cases of PMS, are the artificial chemicals with which modern food and drink are loaded. If these chemicals cause brain swelling in normal men, women, and children, you can see how much more they must add to the brain swelling in a woman suffering from PMS.

As you can see, cellular waste retention causes the brain to swell, which induces the symptoms of PMS. Eliminating this swelling through sweat, urine, or tears, causes the PMS to get better.

Eliminating foods that contain synthetic chemicals and artificial ingredients from the diet is the only way to permanently decrease the severity of the symptoms of PMS. This is accomplished by increasing water intake and eliminating junk food and carbonated drinks from your diet, not just for the PMS days, but all the time.

In other words, swollen brains induce abnormal, emotional, irrational behavior. Normal, non-swollen brains ensure their owner will have normal, healthy behavior and a good, even-tempered personality. Swollen brains are more common in our society than you might think.

Prevent the Big C: Cancer!

Physicians are always telling everyone to avoid carcinogens, and this is certainly good advice. But as the world is so full of cancer-causing agents, the actual fact is that one *can't* avoid all of them all of the time.

People think that if they lived in more primitive times, there wouldn't be so many cases of cancer. Maybe not—people didn't live very long then. There were carcinogens even for cave dwellers; there was always smoke from the continuous fire, burnt meat was as cancer-causing then as today. They used cooking rocks, getting them hot in the fire, then adding the hot rocks to a pot of soup, adding to the soup any radioactivity or harmful chemicals which happened to be in the rocks they chose. Their primitive medicine men mixed concoctions of who-knows-what for almost any ailment. They spent a great deal of time in the sun, so skin cancer must have been common in those days, even if the ozone layer was still intact.

No, getting in your time machine and going back in history would not be the best way to prevent cancer.

About 10% of all deaths in the U.S.A. are due to cancer. This disease is so dreaded, that anyone contracting cancer also has to fight a tremendous psychological burden of worry and fear.

So often we read in the headlines that a researcher has found a new drug which fights cancer better than previous drugs. They say it has a 'promising future', but years go by and the rate of deaths by cancer gets higher. The medical industry may win a few battles but is still losing the war against cancer.

There are already over 2,000 known carcinogens and the list is growing. Among them, about 200 have so far been proven to induce cancer in humans. Some chemicals such as cigarette smoke, asbestos, nickel compounds, and chromium compounds are known to cause lung cancer.

A group of carcinogens known as aflatoxins are produced by the mold *Aspergillus,* which grows on food such as peanuts and grains. This substance accumulates in the liver, where it is activated and causes liver cancer.

Saccharin, an artificial sweetener that passes into the urine, is suspected of producing bladder cancer.

Heavy metals like arsenic, beryllium, cadmium, lead, and nickel are also associated with some specific cancers, beryllium with bone cancer and lead with kidney cancer, leukemia, and bowel cancer.

Obviously, avoiding cancer-causing chemicals is what we should all try to do. However, we are constantly, without our knowledge, ingesting carcinogens by mouth, inhaling them into our lungs, and absorbing them through the skin.

We simply can't avoid them completely. We are certainly able, however, to dilute the concentration of carcinogens to the level where they cannot induce cancer. By drinking proper quantities of water we can quickly expel the carcinogens out of our bodies by urinating, defecating, and sweating.

People believe wrongly that drinking liquid is the same as drinking water. They are totally different. Only clean, pure water can dilute the contaminates successfully. I realize I stress water-drinking throughout this book, but cell cleansing is the basis of all the Chunging rules and exercises.

Many ingredients of commercial soft drinks may not be carcinogenic when they are added to the soda pop, but it is certainly possible that they could turn into carcinogens after they are metabolized in the body's cells.

Researchers believe a few undetectable tiny cancer cells frequently develop in everyone due to carcinogens in the human body. Fortunately, the body has a strong defense mechanism which kills these cancer cells quickly before they have a chance to proliferate. But if there were too many cancer cells or if the body's defense is down due to overuse, those cancer cells may grow and form malignant tumors. By drinking water, diluting concentrated carcinogens, and washing them away, you can ensure that you have fewer new abnormal cells and you won't overtax your body's defense.

For better understanding, let's say Miss A and Miss B each ingest a miniscule amount of a carcinogenic substance. This carcinogen acts upon 100 cells in the body causing them to become abnormal. This is a small number compared to the body's one hundred trillion total cells.

The immune system would start to destroy these abnormal cells almost immediately. Our defense mechanism tries to kill atypical cells before they have a chance to divide and grow.

If Miss A has bad habits (drinks very little water, doesn't exercise enough to sweat, has poor bowel habits, eats junk food, lets herself get run down, smokes) and Miss B has good habits, Miss B's system will be able to handle this danger much better than Miss A's body.

Miss B is drinking enough water to quickly wash away the waste products and excrete them entirely in feces and urine, remove some waste in sweat, and not add to the problem by eating more junk. Her immune system will, in all probability, be able to kill every abnormal cell and she will avoid cancer.

In Miss A's case, however, it is unlikely that all 100 abnormal cells will be able to be killed before at least a few can divide. Miss A is much more likely to develop the dreaded Big C.

I have not met a non-smoking person in the last ten years who developed cancer if they drank six glasses of water a day, moved their bowels every day, exercised and sweated regularly, and avoided large quantities of salt. In these same ten years, I have seen many persons who are not practicing these good habits develop cancer and other incurable diseases under the age of fifty.

Many people with a family history of cancer live in fear of developing cancer. They say "my father died of colon cancer," or "my mother died of breast cancer," or talk of some other relative who developed cancer. Many people have been told by their doctors that they have a higher chance of developing cancer than if it didn't "run in their family." Most people believe that cancer has strong familial tendencies.

Even if you did inherit genes which could predispose you to cancer, *you did not inherit cancer.* Without exposure to concentrated carcinogens, without exhausting your body's defenses, without allowing waste to accumulate in your body, your genes will not cause your cells to become cancerous.

Since it is impossible to totally avoid carcinogens, please dilute cancer-causing substances with water. Wash away any carcinogens you may have ingested by drinking enough water and by keeping your body healthy through exercise and good bowel habits. Create the conditions within your body which allow the body to kill any abnormal cells which happen to form. This is how to prevent cancer.

The human body is almost all water. Without water, the whole body is a handful of ash. In other words, the human body is a 'water bag'. Even the bag is composed of water. To remain in good health, this water bag must constantly expel contaminated, dirty water, and then be refilled with fresh, clean water.

Coffee, tea, and carbonated beverages are nothing more than chemically contaminated, non-oxygenated, dirty water. Only fresh, clean water will clean your cells.

Are there antidotes for carcinogens? Perhaps vitamins and minerals fulfill this role in a healthy body. At the very least, a sufficient amount of these essential chemicals may set the stage for the immune system to take care of the body properly. There is some evidence that vitamins A, C, and E protect the body from free radical oxygen which causes some cancers.

In my opinion, the waste products from anaerobic metabolism and metabolic error within human cells can also produce carcinogens. For this reason, it is important not to induce a hypoxic state (lack of oxygen) by exercising or working your body to the point of shortness of breath.

If you are already afflicted with cancer:

1. Drink six to ten eight-ounce glasses of water daily, depending on your size.

2. Do Breath Chunging daily. Read the chapter on Breath Chunging to understand why this is important.

3. Start doing basic Chunging exercises to build up your immune system and sweat regularly.

4. Avoid all soda drinks and caffeine products, and minimize salt intake.

5. Move your bowels at least once a day, preferably three times a day after each meal.

6. Meditate. There is much evidence that meditation is helpful in fighting disease.

7. Carefully take all the cancer-treating medications and vitamins which your physician gives you.

These things will certainly increase your chance of survival once you have cancer. If you don't have cancer, please follow the first six of the preceding steps to minimize your chances of ever getting it.

On Tiredness

Most people know what makes them tired—usually too much work, or not enough sleep or rest.

You feel tired when your supply of nutrients is exhausted or when an excess of waste is accumulated. Under these circumstances, your cells cannot work properly, and the cumulative effect on the body is perceived as tiredness. Tiredness might be considered to be pain on a cellular level. Certainly the next step beyond muscular tiredness is muscular pain.

When you rest or sleep, your blood supplies nutrition to your cells and carries away accumulated waste. When this process is finished, the feeling of exhaustion disappears. You wake up refreshed. Armed with this understanding, consider this:

> 1. A person who supplies the proper amount of oxygen to his cells will help his cells 'burn' his nutrients completely, producing less waste, making him less tired than a person who does not get enough oxygen to his cells.

2. A person who eats food that can be easily metabolized, leaving less waste, will be less tired than a person who does not eat this type of food.

3. A person who attempts to wash away his cellular waste using only coffee, tea, so-called fruit juice drinks, and soft drinks will be much more tired than a person who drinks a proper amount of clean water.

4. A person who has proper resting and sleeping habits will be less tired than a person who does not.

The Most Frequent Complaint

Tiredness is one of the most frequent complaints of patients when they visit their physician.

Patients who suffer from persistent tiredness ask their doctor the name of the disease from which they are suffering and request that he give them drugs that will make them feel better instantly.

On most occasions doctors are unable to come up with a single name for the disease. After many expensive, sophisticated diagnostic tests, the test results are usually found to be within the normal range. Consequently, there is no clear-cut indication to prescribe a drug for this malady.

When doctors don't know what the mechanics of an illness are, they like to use the word 'syndrome', which means a group of symptoms which characterize a particular disease. So they have come up with the name 'Chronic Fatigue

Syndrome'. With this diagnosis, the patient is happy to have a name for the tired feeling so they can tell their family and employer. The fact is that there is no drug which the doctor can give to his patient which cures this syndrome. They can only advise their patient to rest for weeks and months. Alternatively, they may prescribe something they are sure won't hurt them, like vitamins. "Get more exercise" is also a common prescription, but this is the last thing a tired person wants to hear.

I have my share of patients who arrive at my office after having been diagnosed by another physician as suffering from so-called Chronic Fatigue Syndrome. Since these patients do not recover quickly from this condition of tiredness, they tend to seek a second and third opinion, going from doctor to doctor.

Recently, researchers have thought that a virus is the cause of the disease, but they are not sure. As this is outside my field of study, I have no opinion as to the validity of this as a cause in a true case of Chronic Fatigue Syndrome. People who really have this disease can't function at all; they cannot even get out of bed.

I can only conclude that my patients complaining of tiredness but who are not totally incapacitated by it do not really have Chronic Fatigue Syndrome. Tiredness is a symptom. Just because tiredness may not be linked to a specific disease, however, does not make each case of tiredness any less important to me as a physician, nor does the degree of tiredness the patient is experiencing. I always treat tiredness as a very important symptom. No one wants to go dragging through life—tired all the time and complaining about it.

As I studied tiredness, I found it to be a complex set of problems. A description of the exact way the tiredness effects the patient is important in searching for clues. A person who feels tired 'behind the eyes' probably has totally different problems from a person who is so tired that they tingle all over. Obtaining a history and analyzing the exact way or ways in which the patient feels tired is the first step in analyzing the problem.

Allergies, for instance, cannot be overlooked in searching for a solution to tiredness. A person with allergies may have different forms of tiredness on different days.

Hypothyroidism and anemia are other common causes of the symptom of tiredness. A diabetic also complains of tiredness, as do people with tuberculosis and AIDS. In fact, in almost every disease, people complain of tiredness.

After I applied my own analysis of the mechanism of the symptom 'tiredness' I started to win the fight against it. I want to share my thoughts on this.

First you have to understand muscle tiredness. A person who is lifting a heavy weight may have no difficulty the first few times. After continuing this lifting motion, he will soon experience muscle tiredness, and if he keeps on lifting, he will finally become unable to move. In order to work, muscles have to metabolize nutrients to produce energy. This metabolism produces waste. So, if he exhausted readily available nutrients or energy sources and did not allow time for his muscles to recover before he made them do more work, his muscle cells will become saturated with waste from their own metabolism.

Accumulation of the muscle's metabolic waste is the major cause of muscle tiredness. After the muscles are rested, the blood carries away the waste and the muscle recovers its strength again.

The same goes for the whole body. When a person states that he is tired, it means his body is saturated with metabolic wastes.

My observation is that people who think they suffer from this syndrome have at least several of the following factors:

1. Most of them are not drinking enough water.

2. They frequently suffer from constipation.

3. They drink a lot of soda pop, coffee, or junk drinks.

4. They hate to exercise, and they rarely sweat. If they do exercise, sweat does not come easily.

5. They have an improper sleeping pattern.

6. They eat large quantities of food, especially fat and protein.

7. They may be in a state of depression.

If you analyze these factors, you can see that each one can make more waste in the body.

1. Low water intake makes it difficult for wastes to be expelled from the body.

2. Fewer bowel movements mean that more waste remains somewhere in the system. Not having a bowel movement for three days would be the same as using, but not flushing the toilet for three days. If you continued to flush only occasionally, the whole house would smell. There are many young people who say "I never move my bowels more than twice a week, and I never have any problems." Although they may have no problems at their present age, just wait until they get over fifty. They *will* have problems!

3. The more junk drinks you have, the more junk chemicals stay in your body. Unlike the proverbial computer slogan, "trash in, trash out," some small traces of all the preservatives and other unnatural chemicals do remain in the body.

4. The human body is like a washer. If you put water in with your clothes in a washer, and then drain it right out again, the clothes will still be dirty. Even if you were washing clothes in a clear stream, in order to be cleaned properly, the clothes have to be agitated, twisted, and squished to expel the dirt. Even primitive people know that. Exercise does the same thing for the body.

Using compression and expansion is the only way the body can be properly cleansed. I call this 'active cleansing'. But you must remember that exercise itself produces metabolic waste. That is why it is so important to pursue 'proper' exercise, which I will discuss in a later chapter. Improper or excessive exercise can be harmful.

5. During sleep, the human body performs 'passive cleansing'. Allowing enough hours of restful sleep is essential to allow the body to clean up its act each night.

6. If you eat a large volume of food, more waste is produced.

7. Depression and a bad attitude are symptoms of fatigue rather than a cause of the problem. Accumulation of excessive waste in the human body causes chemical changes in the brain which bring about the feeling of depression.

Then why do researchers find viruses in the person who suffers from true Chronic Fatigue Syndrome? Here is my explanation. Viruses are opportunists. They only induce disease when cells, tissues, and organs are unnecessarily saturated with body waste. For example:

1. Fever blisters (due to the herpes simplex virus) often appear only when a person gets very tired and sick (saturated with waste). When the person has a physically good feeling (little waste in the body), fever blisters almost never appear.

2. People get the flu when they are exhausted. It is difficult for really healthy persons to get the flu.

I believe that many human cells host a few viruses all the time. The viruses don't harm the cells, they are just dormant when the cells are clean. When the cells become contaminated with an excess of waste, the viruses are activated and multiply, manifesting their characteristic harmful effects. It is logical to me that this is the reason researchers find viruses in people who suffer from Chronic Fatigue Syndrome.

It is also my belief that a person who only carries the dormant virus cannot infect a healthy person, just as a person who suffers from recurrent fever blisters, cannot, as a rule, infect others when the blisters are in remission. I also believe that healthy and clean cells cannot easily be infected by most viruses even through direct contact. That is why some people who are exposed to a viral disease like fever blisters, genital herpes, and even HIV are not infected by the active virus.

Keep your body clean inside and out and you won't feel tired *and* you will be protected from viral disease.

Understanding Arthritis

Health books disagree over which parts of the body first show signs of aging. Some say it starts with the feet. Others claim aging starts in the back, still others say the eyes.

To me, it seems logical that aging must start in those parts of the body where the least amount of blood circulates. Those are the hardest places for the body to supply with nutrition and oxygen. Accumulation of waste is also more of a problem in those areas, because it is more difficult for the body to cleanse those parts of waste. As I explained before, the biggest factor in aging is the accumulation of waste in the cells.

That is why I believe that joints are the first places where aging becomes obvious. This aging manifests itself as a lessening in your range of joint motion.

At birth, you have the widest range of joint motion. As you age, some joints just won't move as far as they did in the past. Even a young child is not as flexible as a baby. So, the process continues through youth; by high school, only a few girls are still flexible enough to do the splits. Not many high school boys can do the Russian deep-knee bend dance, either, so you can see that a great amount of flexibility is already lost by both sexes by the teen age years.

The aging person finds it increasingly difficult to move over the entire range of the joint's motion. Because of that, they tend to move each joint less than they did before and less far. This makes them feel increasingly stiff as they age, and in fact, they are not as flexible as when they were younger.

It is important to understand why this limitation of motion occurs.

Joints are meeting places between two or more bones. Usually, smooth cartilage covers the bones within the joint. Joints are surrounded and immersed in a protein fluid called senovial fluid (pronounced *sen o' vee al*), which lubricates the joints. Cartilage is composed of cells called *chondrocytes.*

Cartilage has no blood vessels. It must get its oxygen and nutrition from the blood supply of the bone to which it is attached. Since there is no blood supply or blood vessel to drain waste, the chondrocytes take in nutrition and expel waste through the process of diffusion and osmosis.

Unfortunately, cleansing by diffusion and osmosis are not sufficient to keep the chondrocytes healthy and clean. Cartilage needs frequent expansion to draw nutrients from the bones and then compression to expel the waste. When the cartilage is not properly compressed and expanded by movement, the cartilage becomes malnourished and starts accumulating waste within its cells.

Most often this unhealthy situation begins to develop on the periphery of the cartilage because the edge of the cartilage is only compressed when the joint moves in its full range. However, the daily activity of most adults does not require the full range of motion. When the cells (chondrocytes) on the edge of the joints start accumulating waste inside the cells, the first symptoms of arthritis appear.

This type of arthritis (rheumatoid) is different than osteoarthritis which is the result of trauma of the joint. Doctors call this rheumatoid condition an auto-immune disease, which means that the body's defense system fights against its own cells. So far, physicians and researchers have been unable to find the cause of this type of auto-immune disease. Some physicians believe this mechanism is due to a defective immune system in the body. Some think it is caused by a virus.

Since daily life does not often require full range of motion of the joints, only the center part of the cartilage of one bone end rubs only the center of the opposite joint surface. Therefore, insufficient compression and expansion takes place on the edges of the cartilage. This leads to the accumulation of waste within the chondrocytes towards the margin of the joint.

This waste-containing cartilage continues to thicken and loses its elasticity. These contaminated cells start malfunctioning. Malfunctioning cells trigger the body's immune system into action which induces inflammation around the joint. This causes pain and swelling, which are the first signs of arthritis.

A person suffering from arthritis often feels severe pain in his joints. These joints begin to swell until they are so deformed that they are immovable. Usually only a few select joints have this trouble. Just as individual people have different tolerance levels, individual joints have different tolerances toward the build-up of toxic chemicals in the cartilage. Weak and sensitive joints become more easily diseased. At different times, one person may experience arthritis pain in different joints.

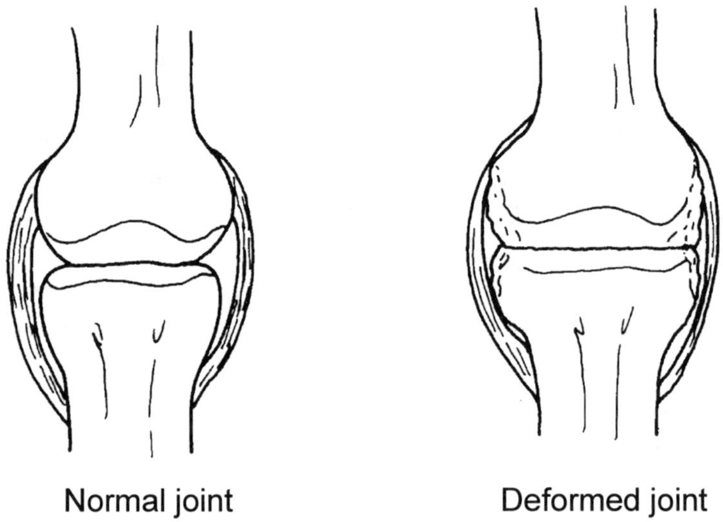

A joint is composed of billions of cells. When a joint cell is weakened, its ability to eliminate its waste products is also lessened. As more waste collects, the joint becomes weaker.

An elaborate immune system protects the body. When a germ enters the human body, the immune system sends soldiers to combat that germ. The immune system calls for an increased supply of blood cells to hasten to the spot and eliminate the contamination. Most of the time, the immune system can handle the job of attacking and eliminating bacteria and viruses which are foreign to the body.

But in rheumatoid arthritis, the cause of the disease mechanism is the body's own contaminated cells. Once the body's cells themselves become diseased, the immune system becomes confused as to what is waste material and what are the body's own cells. The white blood cells, the white knights of the kingdom of the body, are not properly equipped to make this distinction. Diseased cells are interpreted as invading dragons, and the knights set out to destroy them.

It is like the difference between the American army during wartime and local law enforcement's battle against crime. The Armed Forces can wipe out an outside enemy (attacking bacteria) better than the law can deal with crimes perpetrated by its own citizens (the diseased body's own cells). The law can do some of the job—but not nearly enough. It is hard to identify all the bad guys. When it does identify bad guys who are citizens, the law doesn't kill them, it puts them in jail.

The human body has a mechanism similar to jailing. It is called fibrosis. The body has the power to cover up sick cells, effectively isolating sick cells instead of killing them. When the condition persists, fibrosis continues its build-up and the affected area gets bulky, and the joint becomes deformed.

Soon, calcium begins to be deposited near the center of this fibrosis. Pain and stiffness make the patient tend to move even less. The expansion and contraction of the joint is lessened as motion is restricted, thus accentuating the problem.

To better understand this mechanism, consider the following example. If a house were attacked by outsiders, all the members of that household would unite to fight to eliminate them. But if one member of that family became lazy and obnoxious, disturbing everyone, the members of the family might *want* to throw the miscreant out, but family ties may prevent them from doing so. This is the problem the auto-immune system faces. Your own cells are 'family'.

In order to combat arthritis, doctors give their patients aspirin, ibuprofen, and cortisone. Aspirin and ibuprofen have an anti-inflammatory function and reduce pain.

Cortisone also reduces the pain, and sometimes the effects seem almost miraculous. But cortisone works differently from aspirin. It temporarily stops the immune system from functioning. In this way, the body can temporarily ignore the problem although the disease is still present. If the dysfunction of the immune system were confined to the affected joint only, perhaps the application of cortisone would be less harmful. This is not the case, as cortisone actually shuts down the immune system for the entire body, making the patient more susceptible to any other disease that comes along.

I am opposed to the continued use of cortisone for this reason, but it is a useful drug when injected into a joint which is having an acute arthritic attack. It eases the pain and makes the joint move more smoothly, thus allowing the patient to continue more normal movements and get more exercise.

Although men also get arthritis, it is more common in women because women don't move as much as men. Men tend to have more osteoarthritis caused by trauma to the joints.

Women have more rheumatoid arthritis and auto-immune disease than men due to limited full range motion of joints and physical inactivity. Therefore, women have less active cleansing of the cells within the joints. In the last fifty years, women's physical activity has been increasing, and fortunately, the rate of women's arthritis has been decreasing.

When Joint Pain Develops

When joint pain develops, you must move your joints slowly over their full range of motion. Keep in mind that you must progress slowly, only stretching your joints until you feel discomfort. Soon, you will be able to move your joints over their entire, natural range by developing the healthy elasticity of your joints. Slow and steady movement of the joints through their entire range of motion allows expansion and compression of the cartilage. To keep the cartilage elastic, the cartilage cells, which have no blood supply of their own, must be able to cleanse the waste products out of the cell bodies. Compression and expansion removes the waste.

Researchers occasionally claim viral infection as a cause of arthritis, but I believe that it is not a cause but a result: viruses will always appear anywhere there are dirty cells.

Hand Chunging

Hand Chunging promotes circulation to the joints of the hand, aids in elimination of waste products, and keeps your fingers flexible and pain free. To prevent arthritis and cure existing arthritic conditions I recommend the following exercises:

> Step 1. Rotate each joint of each finger individually through its full range of motion using your other hand.

You may feel some minor pain, but as long as you move slowly, you will not cause any damage.

Step 2. Massage every joint in both hands with your opposing index and middle finger and thumb until your joints feel warm.

Step 3. Compress and rub your palms with your thumbs.

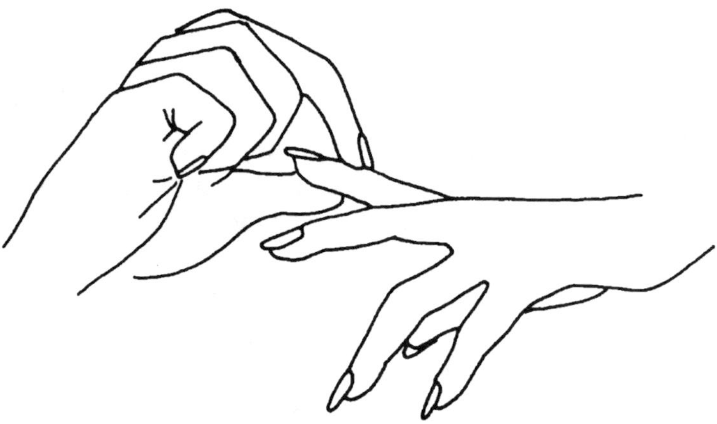

Joint pain is one of the most frequent and debilitating expressions of aging. By the age of sixty-five, about 80% of the population has some arthritic disorder.

These three steps for Hand Chunging can be done any time, anyplace. Do these simple hand exercises watching television, or while you are waiting for the toast to pop up. Exercises like Hand Chunging can prevent arthritic pain, but only if you do the gentle movements frequently.

Gaining Weight is Normal

When you see women in Greek sculpture or Renaissance paintings, they are not the angular fashion model figures we now see in magazines. They were created using real women, normal women as their ideal; well-padded, curving women with a little layer of fat. Nothing much has changed over the centuries. Gaining weight as we grow older is normal.

You, too, should use real people as models for your ideal figure—not the freaks in the high fashion magazines. Have you noticed that most women who are perfectly healthy look nothing like the skinny giants seen in *Vogue*? Very few healthy woman are skin and bones.

Losing weight easily or keeping it off after you lose it *is abnormal.* If 100 women lose fifteen pounds, only three of them will be able to keep it off. Most of them will gain it back—and gain double the pounds lost in just a few years.

Women in their twenties and thirties may, with exercise and moderation, remain slim, but only the most determined can maintain that weight into their forties and fifties.

Of the few who remain slender half a century, most will begin to gain after fifty. Just as people tend to lose weight in really old age, they gain in midlife. This is normal and healthy.

Dieting Doesn't Work

Kathy is a thirty-eight year old registered nurse. She is five feet seven inches tall and weighs 262 pounds. She has two sisters who weigh 150 and 155 pounds. Kathy is an intelligent, energetic worker who is very dedicated in the care of her patients. She is an excellent R.N.

Kathy has been involved with different diet programs throughout her life but she hasn't solved her weight problem.

In order to understand Kathy's weight problem, we must take a close look at her weight history. Kathy weighed eight pounds ten ounces at birth. In her preteen years, she was healthy, slightly overweight, but not fat. When Kathy was eleven years old, she was the tallest girl in her class (5'2") and weighed 150 pounds. Her parents encouraged her to eat less. In six months, Kathy lost five pounds.

When Kathy was fifteen, she weighed 185 pounds. In order to reduce her weight, her family doctor placed Kathy on a 1,000 calories per day diet and also placed her on a thyroid compound which increases metabolism, which, in turn, burns fat more quickly. He also prescribed water pills. In four months, Kathy lost forty pounds.

This result was short-lived. At age seventeen, weighing 200, Kathy once again went on a diet, on the recommendation of the nursing school that interviewed her. Using the same diet as before, (1,000 calories per day, thyroid supplement and water pills), Kathy reduced her weight to 145 pounds.

By the time Kathy was 21, she weighed 200 pounds again. It was the year she graduated from nursing school and her doctor placed her on a fasting diet. Every other week, Kathy would fast. In four months, Kathy had lost 65 pounds: she then weighed 135 pounds.

Kathy tried several other diets after that, and each time, the results were the same. She would lose weight for three or four months, but, time after time, she would gain all, if not more of the weight back. In 1982, at the age of 30, Kathy weighed 250 pounds. At this time, a close friend of hers was going to get married, so she decided to go on another diet for the wedding. This time, Kathy tried a health food diet and lost 50 pounds. During her stringent diet, she would not even go to any social gathering for fear of ruining her diet.

In 1990, at 38 years of age, Kathy weighed at least 262 pounds. She refused to weigh herself since she started gaining weight again. She had become so discouraged with her weight that she is seriously considering returning to the liquid diet system.

Judging from her weight history, returning to any of her old diets seems ludicrous. But Kathy did just that. Why? Is it because of some lack of willpower on Kathy's part? No, Kathy is a very strong-willed woman. Once she chose a diet program, she would continue on that program with all her heart. She would lose weight until she reached her target weight. She (and the diet plans) called this success.

Weight and Willpower

Lack of willpower is *not* the reason some people are overweight. People who are able to go on diets year after year *have* willpower—or they wouldn't be successful in losing the weight they do manage to lose.

Human beings supposedly learn from past experience. If they met with success in the past, like Kathy, they will continue with the same program. If they met with failure, they will usually try the same program once or twice more before moving on to a new weight loss system. Even a chimpanzee that sees a banana hanging from the ceiling will only try to leap and grab it a few times. After the chimp realizes that he cannot reach the banana, he will pile boxes underneath the banana until he can reach the fruit.

So why doesn't the overweight woman ever realize that lack of willpower is not the reason for gaining weight back after she once lost it? How many times do they have to go through this before they realize that the diet programs don't really work? Why can't Kathy, an intelligent woman, realize that returning to her old diet will not work for her this time since it only temporarily worked for her in the past?

Kathy has been brainwashed. Throughout her life, society has unkindly bombarded her with the message, "lose weight, you are fat, fat, fat." The media, through television, magazines, and even junk mail has been telling her that she must lose weight in order to be attractive and happy and that the only way to lose weight is *their* way. The proof that commercial diet programs don't work on a permanent basis is that their customers keep coming back periodically. Kathy will probably gain back the weight she loses in their program this time, too. I believe that the media and society have been giving Kathy the wrong message because *losing the weight is not the real problem.*

The real problem is keeping weight off once you lose it—something diets can't do for you.

The Reason a Fat Person is Fat

To understand why a person becomes fat, you must first understand the main flow of fat. There are two ways nutrients in the body could be metabolized—let's call them two 'channels'—which influence whether or not a person will gain weight. I call them the Dieting Channel and the Chunger Channel.

- If a person metabolizes through the Dieting Channel, the outcome is predictable. The person will increasingly become heavier and fatter within a few years following weight reduction by dieting.

- If a person metabolizes through the Chunger Channel, she will be able to maintain her weight, and to eventually lose weight, if that is desired.

Each of these Channels has six main factors, and they are interconnected. A change in one causes changes in the others.

I have outlined these ideas in the chart on the next page. This will show more graphically why dieting doesn't work.

The Flow of Fat

The Dieting Channel	The Chunger Channel
1. The person craves and eats fattier food.	1. The Chunger person desires and eats less fatty food.
2. Intestines absorb more nutrition into the blood.	2. Intestines absorb less nutrition into the blood.

Once in the blood, these absorbed nutrients have two destinies—they can be stored or they can be spent. If nutrients get into the cells, the cells have to cope with it. One way cells handle extra nutrients is to store the extra calories as fat. The fat is stored in fat cells. People who have lost weight by dieting in the past have more and larger fat storage capacity in the fat cells.

The Dieting Channel	The Chunger Channel
3. Stores more in fat cells.	3. Uses more in working cells.
4. Nutrients are metabolized by the cells slowly, creating more fat.	4. More nutrients are metabolized by the cells quickly and are less likely to turn into fat.

The main end product of metabolism is water and carbon dioxide. The person who gets water and carbon dioxide out of the body faster produces less fat. These end products are eliminated by urination, sweating, and breathing.

The Dieting Channel	The Chunger Channel
5. Less water intake, less output. Lack of water slows down metabolism.	5. Increased water consumption moves waste out of body faster and more thoroughly.
6. Exhaling less carbon dioxide slows down metabolism.	6. Proper elimination of carbon dioxide activates cell metabolism.

In other words, ingested food is digested, then absorbed into the blood as nutrients. Then the circulatory system distributes it to the body cells.

If there are more nutrients than the body cells need, the nutrients are stored as fat in the fat cells until it is needed by the working cells. The working cells use these nutrients to accomplish work. In this process, the nutrients are mainly turned into carbon dioxide and water.

As I said before, there are six main factors (besides heredity) in deciding who will be fat and who will be thin. When you restrict food intake, you are restricting only one of these factors and *activating* the other factors such as:

1. The absorption of more nutrients from intestines.

2. The storing of more fat in the fat cells.

3. A slowing down of the metabolism of the cells.

Suppressing this one factor, diet, may allow a person to lose weight temporarily, but as it activates other factors, it makes the person get fatter in the future. There are additional factors, such as attitude,which I will mention later.

Don't be proud if you have lost weight quickly by dieting. You are only preparing yourself to be a fatter person in the future by increasing the activity of other fat-inducing factors. You are activating a starvation mode which makes your body more efficient for the next year. No matter what method of weight loss dieters use, most will be fatter than before dieting within five years. This is a fact.

Diet commercials show a chubby and fat person before dieting and a trim, fit person who states that they were unhappy before losing their weight. But seldom do you see that same person in their ads five years later. I believe most of them turn obese, a lot fatter than before. And, they will still feel unhappy with themselves.

Kathy is a typical example of the phenomenon: crash dieting causing eventual, even larger, weight gain. You can see many similar examples, maybe including even yourself.

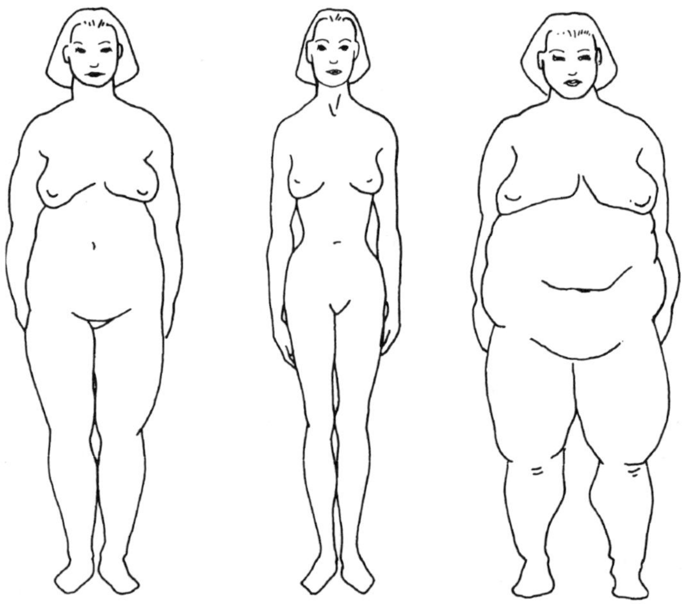

Before dieting After dieting Five years later

Please, wake up! Dieting is not the answer. Please use logic and common sense. A person who weighs 180 pounds now, is steadily gaining weight, and has a good appetite, already has a hard time maintaining her weight at its present level. It is humanly impossible for this same person to lose 50 pounds of weight by dieting, then to maintain her weight at 130 pounds. People who do this almost always gain back the weight and more. Then why do people continue dieting?

Maintain Your Present Weight

A person who is unable to maintain his present weight should not try to lose weight because he will be unable to maintain what he has lost. He will always gain back the weight.

The first step to successfully losing weight is to learn how to maintain your present weight.

It doesn't matter at all what your weight is when you start. Start Maintaining exactly where you are now. This means weighing yourself every morning. Take an average weight of a week or ten days to be your maintenance weight. There will be daily fluctuation. If you are over your Maintaining weight by more than five pounds, try to exercise more, concentrate more on your breathing exercises, and drink more water. You must not eat less nor go on a diet.

There are two reasons to Maintain and continue Maintaining.

First, it takes a long time of Maintaining to change your physiology, about a year to get from the Dieting Channel to the Chunger Channel.

Then, it takes a long time to prove to yourself that you don't have to endlessly gain, that you can successfully Maintain.

To Maintain, you must change the fear of "I am getting fatter" to the confidence of "I am not getting fatter" by proving to both your body and your mind that you have succeeded.

This method does not allow you to deceive yourself. Your body chemistry cannot be fooled. Nor can this process be speeded up—it takes a full year of Maintaining your weight at its present level for these needed body-chemistry changes to become permanent.

Once you have developed the 'confidence' you will witness the 'magic'. Excess fat will start disappearing spontaneously and effortlessly. How? Your body gets out of the Dieting Channel, and into the Chunger Channel.

In the long run, the person who wishes to maintain his present weight will almost always eat less than a person who wishes to lose weight.

This is one of the reasons why a person who truly wishes to maintain or even gain weight will start to lose weight and the person who wishes to lose will end up gaining.

Attitude

I am not a psychologist, but it is obvious to me that a person who believes he is 'good' will tend to do good things. A person who believes he is 'bad' will do harmful things and become worse. Examples of this are found everywhere.

Exactly the same principle applies to weight. People who think they are fat get fatter, while people who think they are thin get thinner or are able to stay slim. I frequently get complaints from people who are overweight. Even though they don't eat, they say, they continue to gain weight. I also get complaints from people who are underweight, saying that, even though they eat constantly, they continue to lose weight.

One of the initial factors that causes a person to become fat is the 'fear' of becoming a fatter person. Fear makes a person eat more by making them nervous. Fear makes them join a diet program, which almost always proves to be devastating.

People who are generally happy and self-confident tend to look more distinguished and appealing than people who suffer from inferiority complexes. Self-confidence shows; their whole body language is different, better. It is the same way with weight.

For example, there are not many obese Asians. Why? When Asians gain weight, their peers appreciate and envy them because in Asian countries, gaining weight is equated with success and wisdom. You may have noticed that all the statues of the Buddha depict him as slightly overweight. This is not seen as unattractive; rather, it is a sign of wisdom and prosperity. Thus, Asians are proud to be 'chubby'.

In Korea, if a married woman is fat, people say she looks like the first daughter-in-law of a rich family—a compliment. If a man gets heavy, they say he looks like a general in the army or the president of a company. When Asians put on a few pounds, they are comfortable with their weight. They don't try to diet. Therefore, their weight remains stable and obesity never becomes a problem.

Another example of attitude affecting weight is one that I see often in my profession as a gynecologist. Many overweight women begin to lose weight or stay the same when they become pregnant. When I ask them if they have been skipping meals or have placed themselves on special diets, most say, no. In fact, most report that they have been eating more than before. Obstetricians usually tell them they should gain two to three pounds a month during pregnancy.

The reason why overweight women often lose weight during pregnancy is because, for the first time in their lives, their peers and family tell them that it is okay to gain weight. Being allowed, even encouraged, to gain weight is a profound psychological burden lifted from their hearts. These women feel comfortable with the shapes of their bodies during pregnancy. That is usually the first time in their lives that they have been freed from the obsession of losing weight. Therefore they are able to maintain or even lose a few pounds.

Human life is never stable. When everything is going well with job, children, spouse, and parents, people find it is easier to maintain lost weight. But when life events cause sadness, anger, and frustration, the amount of food people eat increases. An unhappy person will gain until she weighs as much as she ever did before. But it never stops there; each binge takes them beyond their previous maximum weight.

A final example of attitude affecting weight comes from simply observing obese people. Most obese people range in weight from 200 to 250 pounds. After obese people reach this upper limit, they usually give up in their attempts to lose weight, and having made that psychological concession, their weight begins to stabilize.

Change Your Attitude

Changing your attitude has a long-term effect. Once the change has been made, you will never gain weight again.

An obese person often knows the difference between right eating and wrong eating. If he sees an apple and a slice of cheesecake, he will know that eating the apple would be the right thing to do. However, the obese person will still eat the cheesecake, and probably the apple, too.

What, then, determines whether or not a person will do the 'right thing'? Most people would say that the person who eats the cheesecake lacks willpower. I don't personally believe willpower has anything to do with losing weight. Strong willpower is more likely to make the obese person diet more drastically and lose weight faster, which just sets him up for gaining it back quickly again.

The Obsession to Lose Weight is the Source of Obesity

I cannot stress strongly enough how important your attitude is when it comes to your weight. Once you gain your own self-approval, once you become truly satisfied with the shape of your body, only then will your weight stabilize. In fact, you will even see a slight loss of weight, around a pound every month. This may seem quite slow, but in just one year you will be 10-12 pounds lighter. If you are quite overweight, in five years, you will be 50-60 pounds lighter. *Permanently.*

If you can do this—maintain your current weight for one year—you will positively be able to lose weight—slowly, it is true, but permanently. After maintaining your same weight for one year, the magic starts happening.

Only by changing your basic attitude will you continually be able to choose what is right. In obesity, one of the most important factors in changing attitude is water consumption.

The Chunging Way to Lose Weight

The Chunging way of fighting fat is to make individual body cells clean by eliminating cellular waste and unnecessary nutrients. Again, Chunging concentrates on the cleansing side of physiology, not the supply side like the modern health industry, which concentrates on the amounts and character of food intake. Please refer again to the Flow of Fat chart.

Weight loss by Chunging concentrates on how to eliminate carbon dioxide and water. Without the proper elimination of these waste products, the cells cannot properly metabolize nutrients. When a chimney is blocked, the fireplace can't burn wood efficiently. If the chimney is wide open and the smoke flows well, the fire burns much faster, and can burn more wood in a shorter time. The same applies to the body. When carbon dioxide is eliminated quickly, cells burn a larger quantity of nutrients in a shorter time.

Carbon dioxide is eliminated by breathing. That is why I keep stressing the importance of proper breathing. Fat people breathe more shallowly and faster than a thin person. They breathe like a person who is ill.

Breath Chunging is deep, long, and slow breathing. See the chapter on breathing for more information.

Many large cities in the Orient have obesity clinics that teach only how to breathe properly as a means of getting rid of body fat. This concept works very well and those clinics are becoming more popular. When obese people come to the clinic they are told to sit in a meditative position, then to practice correct abdominal breathing for thirty minutes to an hour.

On a recent TV documentary, Tibetan monks in winter time put cold, wet blankets on their naked bodies, and sat in a meditation position and breathed properly. Soon steam was coming off them. By breathing properly, they produced more body heat. This is proof of the high rate of metabolism which can be achieved without exercise—by proper breathing only.

What about water, the other end product of metabolism? Water also has to get out of the body to promote better cell metabolism.

The best way to get rid of the water which is a by-product of metabolism is to drink large quantities of water. This shuts off production of an anti-diuretic hormone from the pituitary gland. With less of the anti-diuretic hormone, the kidneys let a large quantity of water out from your body in the form of urine, which will carry with it other waste products. Eventually the body cells get cleaner, and when they do, they can burn off more nutrients faster.

Body cells can burn off nine times more nutrients than their basal rate, given optimum conditions. Why not give yourself those optimal conditions? By breathing properly, drinking water, and doing proper exercise, you can burn off more fat faster. This creates the proper flow of fat. It is obviously better to increase your efficiency at expelling carbon dioxide and water than to become more efficient at storing fat.

Many weight reduction workshops in the U.S.A. encourage their patients to drink large quantities of water without explaining the logical reason behind this. The operators of these clinics have observed that their patients who drink more water get thinner and stay thinner.

The best fat-burning exercises are deep knee-bends and sit-ups. Fat tends to accumulate around inactive muscles. When abdominal muscles become inactive, there is a tendency to develop a potbelly and 'love handles'. Thigh muscles may become inactive, which will induce a fatty rear end. When chin muscles become inactive, double chins develop.

One of the first changes of obesity and aging is fat around the trunk and hip areas. These changes are absolutely preventable by regular sit-up and deep knee-bending exercises. If you already have a pot-belly and fatty hips you can eliminate all this fat by persistent daily sit-ups and deep knee-bending exercises. These exercises are described in other chapters.

The other important change you have to make is to develop good bowel habits. You must move your bowels more than once a day, preferably three times a day. The reason for this is to make food pass through the intestinal tract faster, thus giving the body less time to absorb extra nutrients.

To make your bowels move more frequently, you must ingest adequate quantities of naturally composed fiber. Drink six to ten glasses of water daily, eat fiber-rich meals, and you can easily change your bowel habits. Please refer to the chapter on gastro-intestinal Chunging.

We must consider each cell as a living individual. Just as a person who eats a meal must expel these nutrients one way or another, a cell which receives nutrients from blood must get this ingested nutrient out of the cell quickly. If not, the cell cannot persist in a healthy life. A person expels waste by defecating, urinating, and breathing. A cell expels the utilized nutrients through the work of the body on a cellular level. If there is no activity in the cell, the cell cannot expel its waste.

Fortunately the vital organs of the human body work their own will constantly; they are cleansing themselves all the time. However, the skeletal muscles do not work unless the individual orders them to work. In other words, muscle cells can't defecate and urinate unless you make them. That is why you have to exercise daily. A person who states that "I only exercise once a week" is only expelling waste from his muscles once a week. The stagnant nutrients are as bad as waste, just like undigested and stagnant meals in the stomach are as bad as being constipated.

The Best Exercise to Lose Weight

The most important part of an automobile is the engine. The engine burns gas with the help of oxygen. By doing that, it produces power to move the car. Then where is the engine of a human being? Many say the answer is the heart, so they stress the importance of cardio-vascular exercise. However, the heart is merely a distributor of fuel, a pump that moves the nutrients in the blood, delivers the waste carbon dioxide to the lungs for expulsion, and carries the waste to the kidneys for elimination.

The real engines of the body are the tiny energy generators within each cell, the *mitochondria.*

The mitochondria are called the 'powerhouses' of the cell. because mitochondria are the place where nutrients turn into energy. Without them, cells could not produce energy from nutrients and oxygen. Without mitochondria you cannot burn fat off. In other words, each cell carries the its own fat burners. The number of mitochondria per cell vary from less than one hundred up to as many as several thousand, depending upon the amount of energy required by each cell.

Mitochondria are self-replicative, which means that one mitochondria can form a second one, third one, and so on, whenever there is need in the cell for an increased amount of energy. Just like an auto maker who can increase the number of cylinders in a car to generate more power, more mitochondria consume more fuel. An eight-cylinder car burns more gas than a four-cylinder car.

As you induce more work in the cell by exercise, the cell will create more mitochondria,which eventually burns off more calories at a faster rate.

Humans are able to command the skeletal muscle to perfom work. The largest skeletal muscle cell mass is the thigh muscle. Therefore, deep knee bending exercise with proper breathing is by far the best exercise for fat burning.

Adult Diabetes

The level of glucose in the blood of a healthy person varies at different times of day—but within a normal range. In diabetics, the glucose level in the blood is too high. In a person with diabetes, glucose stays in the blood because not enough of it can get into the cells where it can be metabolized.

In the United States and Western Europe, the disease affects about 16% of the population above age sixty-five. People with diabetes run ten times the risk of the rest of the population of becoming blind and twenty times the risk of being afflicted with gangrene of the feet. Diabetics risk heart and kidney disease, and many other life-threatening conditions.

Diabetes is a terrible disease; it is a disease which forces one to change one's lifestyle drastically. Everyone who doesn't have diabetes should actively work at trying to keep themselves from getting it later in life by following the Chunging To Lower Blood Sugar exercises. Anyone who already has diabetes should also follow my Chunging rules to keep the disease from becoming worse.

Automobiles need gas in their engines to run. Human beings' major fuel is glucose. Cells need glucose to live, to generate heat. A man uses 1600 calories of nutrients per day to survive, that is, to live and to generate heat. A woman uses about 1400 calories a day for this same basic metabolism.

After a healthy person ingests carbohydrates such as sugar and starch, they turn into glucose which flows into the blood and is then distributed by the blood to the body cells. Cells use glucose as fuel to work, live, and produce heat. Glucose leaves the body as carbon dioxide and water after having been oxidized and turned into energy for the body. These waste products are then expelled by exhalation and urination. This is the flow of normal carbohydrate metabolism.

In diabetes, the flow of this chain of events is blocked at the level at which blood glucose enters the cell, believed to be mainly due to lack of insulin in the blood. Since the intestines continue adding glucose to the blood from absorbed nutrients, and this glucose can't go anywhere else, the concentration of glucose in the blood gets higher and higher. This causes a dangerous condition called *hyperglycemia*, which could induce a coma or even death of the patient.

However, nature has its own defense against this condition by making the patient thirsty. Consequently, the patient drinks large quantities of water which dilutes the concentration of glucose in the blood. The patient then expels this excess glucose through the kidneys as glucose or 'sugar' in the urine. That is the reason why a diabetic person both drinks a lot of water and urinates frequently. This defense mechanism reduces the total amount of glucose in blood and body. But it produces neither a permanent solution nor a cure.

Modern Medicine vs. Chunging

Modern medicine focuses again on the supply side, concentrating on diet and nutrition, insulin injections, and drugs which enhance the body's production of insulin. The conventional treatment for diabetes only corrects the level of glucose in the blood by relocating sugar into the cell. This makes the concentration of glucose in the blood lower, but the total amount of glucose in the body remains the same. The excess glucose has only shifted its location from the blood to the cells. At present we are only temporarily relieving the symptoms of the disease by everyday continuous treatment instead of curing the patient who has diabetes.

Modern commercial laboratories are able to check sugar levels in blood and urine by simple tests. Equipment and test kits are available for the patient to make these tests themselves, once the disease is diagnosed. Determining the levels of sugar within the individual cells would be a difficult and costly procedure. So, checking blood sugar levels and prescribing insulin is "the way its done." Period. What they don't know, they assume is okay. *That may not be true.*

The Langerhans cells, which are the producers of insulin, reside in the pancreas which is located in the upper part of the abdominal cavity. As the Langerhans cells may begin to depend on this external source of insulin, the pancreas could become less functional as the disease goes on.

Chunging focuses on the cleansing side, the elimination of excess sugar from the body, which would eventually cure the disease by making the pancreas healthier if the Langerhans cells are still alive. If they are not, the patient is probably too ill to exercise, possibly mortally ill.

To remain healthy, your pancreas must be in working order. To keep it that way, do not overload your system by binging on sugar, which causes extreme overwork by these marvelous cells.

Besides prescribing insulin to fight adult diabetes, doctors also advise their patients to diet and exercise. Nevertheless, most patients fail to follow this advice because they do not understand why they should avoid certain foods or why exercise helps fight diabetes. Also, it is difficult to stick with a diet and exercise all the time, especially as diabetics may feel so rotten. If the patient skips a meal, or exercises without proper nutrition, the patient develops a condition called hypoglycemia (very low blood sugar) which is as dangerous as hyperglycemia (high blood sugar). Hypoglycemia induces shock which, if not treated promptly and correctly, could claim the patient's life.

Let me compare this flow of carbohydrate metabolism in adult diabetes, with the flow of coal through the boiler of a train. The blood glucose is the coal in the coal bin. The insulin acts like the fireman who shovels the coal from the bin into the firebox. The body cell is the firebox where the coal burns. Adult diabetes is like a coal bin loaded with so much coal that it is overflowing the bin and falling off the train.

Inducing a normal level of blood glucose with insulin is like hiring an extra fireman to shovel the coal faster into the firebox so they can empty the coal bin, without considering if the firebox can handle this much extra coal.

As I have described, adult diabetes is a result of the cells' inability to utilize enough glucose within the cell; therefore, the level of glucose within the cell becomes too high. This prevents the cell from accepting more glucose from the blood. In other words, the firebox (cell) cannot burn all the extra coal (sugar) that is shoveled in by the firemen (insulin).

It is *not* the fact that the first fireman (insulin produced in Langerhans cells) was lazy or ineffective. Therefore, hiring the second fireman (insulin injection to supplement insulin produced by the body) to shovel coal (glucose) into the firebox (cell) at a faster rate did not really solve the problem.

But modern medicine only measures the amount of glucose in the blood (coal bin), and pronounces its treatment a success if the blood (coal bin) has the right amount of glucose (coal).

That is why modern medicine is winning only a few battles against adult diabetes. To win the war, we must learn the true anatomy of diabetes. I believe that we must look into the interior of the cell for a real cure. Only quite recently have we begun to understand some of the involved and specialized chemical activities which go on in the world within the cell.

It seems to me that modern medicine is neglecting two aspects of diabetes, and that doctors should consider these questions:

1. What is the effect of forcing large quantities of sugar into the cell with the help of insulin?

2. Why do physicians think that a high blood sugar level has a worse effect on human health than a high level of sugar within the cells?

It may turn out to be just the opposite. In my opinion, the cells are being suffocated from an overload of glucose. Too much glucose may actually be toxic to individual cells. When sugar is in the blood, at least it can easily be eliminated by the kidneys. This is not true when it is stacked up inside the cells.

Most excess glucose is burned (metabolized) in muscle. When stress arises, your body prepares for action by increasing the level of glucose in the blood. Stress induces an elevation of epinephrine, steroids, and thyroid hormones, which in turn increase the level of blood glucose. The mechanism which prepared primitive man for fight or flight is still in working order today. But modern day stress usually does not require your muscles to work. Thus the blood glucose is not utilized, and the glucose level remains high. In our sedentary lives, there is not enough physical work for the muscles to use all the glucose in the cells which the stress has caused. In addition to this, our normal diets are loaded with refined sugar as additives to a wide range of foods, let alone the amount of sugar we ingest as we indulge ourselves with desserts, candies, and drinks.

Eventually, the excess glucose is turned into fat. Diabetics have high cholesterol and high fat levels in the blood, which makes it even more difficult to utilize glucose, because fat also interferes with the transport of blood sugar into cells.

When the muscles are not utilizing all the glucose, the blood glucose level is too high. The pancreas is therefore called upon to produce more insulin than would be needed if the muscles' activity level were higher. The most natural way to eliminate this high glucose level would be to create work for your muscles. Until we solve the complicated mysteries of diabetes, Chunging To Lower Blood Sugar is the best preventive measure for those with the diabetes-prone body build and/or inherited tendencies toward the disease, or for people addicted to sugar.

Break the Vicious Cycle of Diabetes

Break the deadly cycle of diabetes by:

1. Developing muscle mass.

2. Producing muscle work.

This will burn the excess glucose, and through the mechanisms of breathing and urination, expel it from the body in the form of carbon dioxide and water. In this way, you actually eliminate glucose from the body rather than just moving its location from the bloodstream into the cells.

I hope you can see the need to exercise and to breathe properly. I know I stress proper breathing often. Think of it this way: remember that sugar is composed of carbon, hydrogen, and oxygen; sugar metabolizes into water and carbon dioxide. Breathing properly alone, even when *not* exercising, eliminates a surprising amount of excess sugar by greatly increasing the production of carbon dioxide. Carbon dioxide is one of the main waste products of the body. Getting rid of it is often not given much thought and attention by conventional medicine. Breath Chunging exercises are designed to cleanse the body of this waste product efficiently, even when you are at rest or meditating. Breath Chunging is even more efficient when combined with other Chunging exercises.

If there is a disorder of the pancreas which has caused the Langerhans cells to have actually been destroyed, unfortunately, these suggestions won't help. Diabetes often runs in families; however, it well may be that the disease itself is not inherited, but rather the body type which makes one more prone to the disease.

People who have thin legs and a heavy upper body develop adult diabetes more often than those who have heavier thighs and a smaller upper torso. Women who are overweight with large hips and thighs have only a small chance of getting diabetes. If you have the shape most prone to diabetes, or if you have a mild case of diabetes, Chunging to Lower Blood Glucose may make a wonderful difference in your life.

The largest muscle mass in your body is the thigh, which, when being worked, can burn a large quantity of blood glucose. In fact, if you develop a large mass of muscle in your thighs, you will prevent adult diabetes, or if you already have the disease, at least you will prevent the disease from getting worse, which is well worthwhile. Reversing this body shape, so that you have thicker thighs and thinner torso, will prevent

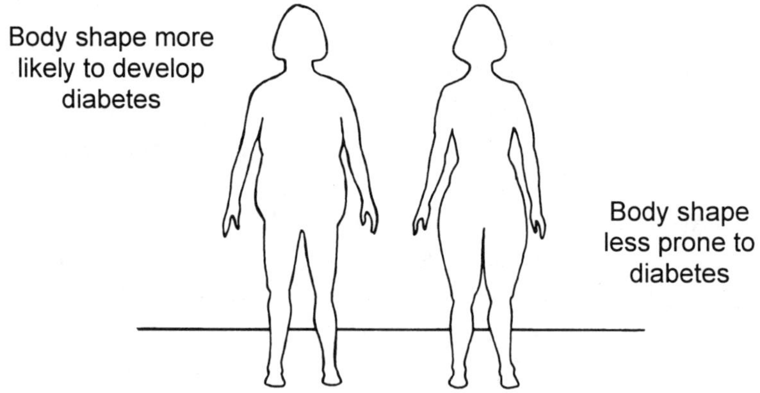

or improve the disease. The importance of maintaining well-developed thigh muscles even into old age should be obvious. Aside from its prevention of diabetes, many other disabilities can be prevented by maintaining good muscle tone.

Chunging To Lower Blood Sugar: Deep Knee Bends

You probably think that working on an exercise bike or rowing machine is a good thigh exercise, and you are right. Walking is excellent, too, but the very *best* thigh exercise of all is doing deep knee bends or squatting. I consider Chunging to Lower Blood Sugar (deep knee bends) one of the most important of all the Chunging exercises.

First, place both hands on top of a desk or on the back of a substantial chair to stabilize yourself. Slowly bend your knees fully, and just as slowly, raise back up until you are in a standing position.

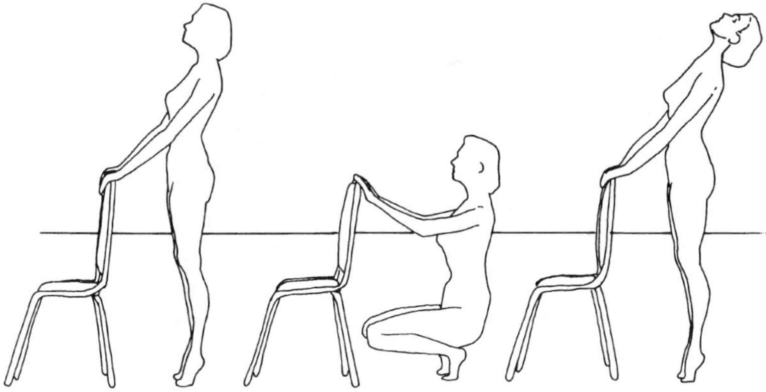

At this point you may hear a cracking noise from your knee joints. As long as you move slowly and don't feel any pain in the knee joint, you will not do any damage. No Chunging exercise should be painful. If you feel actual pain (as opposed to discomfort from muscles you are not used to using), discontinue the exercise.

If, on squatting once, you can't get up again without pulling yourself up with your arms, begin your exercises at that squatting level. Work toward being able to rise to a standing position from a squatting position without the help of your arm muscles. Make the thigh muscles do the work.

Do as many deep knee bends as you can until you feel uncomfortable. If you can only do five deep knee bends or less on your first day, do not become discouraged. Many other people are in the same situation. On the next day, try to increase the number of knee bends by one. Continue to increase the number daily or weekly. When you can do more than ten knee bends comfortably, start the practice of Breath Chunging as part of this exercise: exhaling slowly through your mouth when squatting, and inhaling through your nose while regaining a standing position.

By the time you can do twenty deep knee bends a day without feeling shaky the next day, you will begin to feel strength return to your thighs. If you check your blood sugar level after this exercise, it will be lower. Of course, each person will advance at a different rate.

Don't overdo this exercise at first. If you do too many deep knee bends, you may have trouble going up and down stairs the next day due to stiffening of your leg muscles.

The creaking sounds in your knee may continue. As long as there is no pain or swelling, you are okay. Ignore minor muscle soreness as it will disappear in a few days if you continue this exercise. Knees can be hurt by jarring or twisting, but not by slow bending and stretching. It may take a month before you feel comfortable with deep knee bends.

Deep knee bends are a difficult exercise for most people. Look at it this way:

- A Chunger person can get up again when he or she is on the floor. Thigh muscles should accomplish this.

- At any age, a Chunger person can get up out of a chair without holding on to something. Thigh muscles should do this for you, too.

- Deep knee bends tone the largest and strongest muscle. Strong thigh muscles help prevent diabetes, obesity, and hypertension.

These simple things are pretty basic to life. Yet many people lose this basic ability while they are only in their fifties. Why? Simply because they stop bending at the knees and instead, lean over from the hips to pick up something, rather than squatting like a little child does, when picking up a toy.

Adults lose muscle tone because they can feel the strain when they try to use muscles, and therefore they avoid using them. But muscles are incredible! It takes resolve, but thighs respond to use. They can be rebuilt and strengthened. Older adults who have been doing deep knee bends walk like a young person. They maintain mobility and have confidence that they can continue to care for themselves and their family. These goals are well worth the time and a few muscle aches.

How many deep knee bends a day? As many as you can. Thirty to fifty is enough to keep your thighs strong. The point of deep knee bends is to burn sugar, build muscle, and to exercise joints over their entire range of motion.

Diet for Adult Diabetes

I recommend you follow the diet suggested by the American Diabetic Association.

Fruits, vegetables, and oatmeal contain a mixture of many forms of carbohydrates. Complex carbohydrates do not over-stimulate or damage the pancreas. The best diet for diabetics is composed of beans and bean products (tofu), fish, poultry (without the skin), and fruits and vegetables.

If healthy humans take in more calories than are needed for basic survival, the extra calories have one of three destinies. The best outcome would be that they are consumed by the work of the cells, mostly in the muscles. If it is not metabolized, it will be stored in the body as glycogen stored in the liver, ready to be called into use when needed as fuel, or as fat stored in the fat cells. Once inside the fat cells, the body does not call for it unless other sources of fuel are exhausted.

Author's Note* Juvenile diabetes is quite different from adult diabetes. People who have juvenile diabetes *must* take insulin to control their disease. Insulin is good medicine; it has saved countless lives. However, it must be used properly.

Hypertension

The World Health Organization defines normal blood pressure as below 140 for systolic pressure and 90 for diastolic. Blood pressure means "the force exerted by the blood against any unit area of the vessel wall." When one says that systolic blood pressure is 120 this means that the force exerted is sufficient to push a column of mercury up to a level 120 mm high when the heart is contracting. When diastolic pressure is 80, it means the force pushes the mercury column to 80 mm when the heart is resting.

Hypertension is a sustained elevation of the arterial systolic pressure of 160 or more, or a diastolic pressure of 95 or more. People who have high blood pressure have a greater risk of developing cardiovascular diseases such as heart disease or experiencing strokes.

Blood pressure generally increases slightly with age. Sixty percent of all people over sixty have hypertension. Actually, since the disease does not show any symptoms, the incidence is probably much higher.

Since the blood is contained in a system which is constructed of the blood vessels and the heart, the pressure becomes elevated by two basic causes. The first is an increase in blood volume, known as volume-loading hypertension. The second cause is any constriction of the blood vessels, which is called vaso-constrictor hypertension.

Fortunately, most hypertension is reversible by eliminating these two basic causes.

Volume-Loading Hypertension

This type of hypertension is caused by increased fluid volume in a human body. Since a major portion of the fluid in the human body is salty water, you can induce hypertension by consuming excess salt and water, and you can produce lower blood pressure by eliminating salt and water. That is why the first medicine prescribed by the doctor for hypertension is a diuretic (water pill), the chief function of which is to eliminate salt from the body. This in turn will increase the elimination of water. Most of the time, this alone will return a person's high blood pressure to normal. Although it may correct the problem, the results are short lived, and the person may have to take diuretics regularly to maintain a normal blood pressure for the rest of his life.

The constant use of diuretics can be harmful, because along with the water which is removed from the body through urine, potassium is also lost. Hydrochlorothizide, the most widely used diuretic, minimizes the body's ability to metabolize sugar, and increases levels of cholesterol and fat in the blood.

The same effect of diuretics can be achieved without the side effects of drugs by simply minimizing salt intake and drinking large quantities of water, because water itself is a strong diuretic which eliminates unnecessary body salt and fluid. Again, *drinking water is the answer.*

Vaso-Constrictor Hypertension

A constricted blood vessel induces hypertension, and a dilated blood vessel produces lower blood pressure.

Stress is the major cause of constricted blood vessels because of stress-induced stimulation by the sympathetic nervous system. Stimulating this system elevates blood pressure directly by exciting the heart and blood vessels, and indirectly by the release of epinephrine and norephinephrine from the adrenal gland, which further excites the heart and constricts blood vessels.

Eliminating stress completely is the key but usually that is impossible because so many people today lead a stressful life style. However, you can minimize its effect by utilizing the parasympathetic nervous system, which counteracts stress. I will discuss how to make use of this wonderful system by Parasympathetic Chunging in the following chapter.

Chunging for Hypertension

I would like to introduce two exercises which are very effective in lowering high blood pressure. Even if you are not hypertensive, do this Chunging to prevent hypertension.

Foot Chunging

It has been said that a person who has healthy feet will live a long, healthy life and will almost never get sick. This is very true. The foot is the farthest organ from the brain, heart and lungs. Because of this distance, the foot shows the first signs of dysfunction of the brain, heart, and lungs.

Foot Chunging promotes better circulation in your feet which will make your feet Chunger and will prevent hypertension.

Step 1. Rub your toes individually with your fingers in a rotating motion ten to twenty times.

Step 2. Stretch your legs. While stretching, rub your big toe with your second toe.

Step 3. Hit the middle of your soles gently with your fist a hundred times.

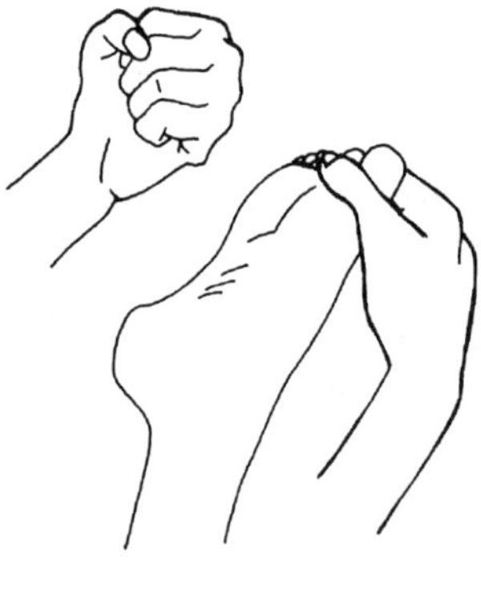

Try to practice this exercise at least once a day. If you can do more, it's a good idea. Take your shoes off and put your feet up while you are watching television; do your Foot Chunging during the commercials instead of dashing out to the kitchen for snacks.

The longest and largest artery is the artery from the heart to the toes. This artery is the Mississippi River of the body. If this river flows well, all its tributaries flow well. If the arteries flow well, hypertension cannot develop.

Toes are the farthest part of the body from the heart, and blood pressure is lower when it reaches to the toes. Also, it is not so easy for blood to flow through the toes. When toes cannot get sufficient blood, the heart pumps harder and stronger to increase its pressure to supply adequate blood to these pitiful organs. In other words, the circulation at the toes and feet affect blood pressure, and you can lower your blood pressure by making your toes and feet have smooth circulation.

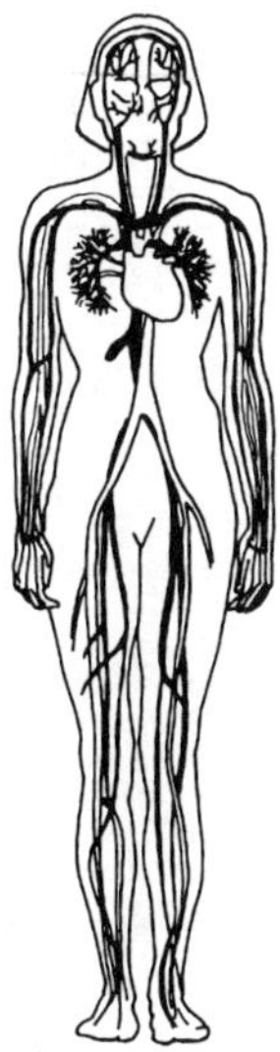

If socks or garters restrict the flow of blood to the feet, they also restrict the blood going back to the heart.

People who have heart, kidney, and lung problems often have swollen feet. Diabetics who have deteriorating nerves and blood vessels are often afflicted with inflammation, infection, and gangrene of their toes and feet. In addition, smokers who develop nicotine toxicity often develop gangrene in their toes.

There are practitioners who claim they can cure diseases by manipulation or massaging of the feet. Also, acupuncturists have found that the feet contain approximately one fourth of the total amount of acupoints on the body. (Acupoints are the points on the body where acupuncturists insert needles which eliminate symptoms of diseases and, often, cure diseases.)

When the blood in the arteries reaches the toes, it goes through smaller and smaller arteries until it reaches capillaries, which are the tiniest blood vessels. The capillaries connect to the small veins, which become larger and larger as the blood goes toward the heart.

Thermo-regulating Capillary Exercise

As you see in the following picture, the smallest artery (arteriole) goes through a capillary vessel before it comes into the smallest vein (venule). Human blood pressure has to be high enough to push blood all the way through the arteriole. A person must keep the structure of this peripheral vessel healthy so that the blood flows smoothly. This structure is made of very fine smooth muscle which dilates when hot and constricts when cold.

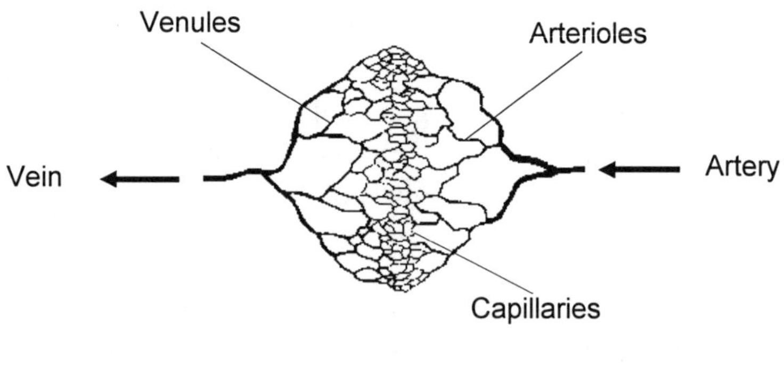

How blood travels from the arteries to the veins

An American traveler, visiting an Oriental public bath house, will witness strange behavior in many Asians. A few Asians sit in a deep tub of very hot water until their skin heats up and turns red. This redness means their capillary vessels are dilated in full. Then they abruptly jump into very cold water in a nearby tub. They stay in the cold water until their skin looks like the skin of a plucked goose. This sudden chilling means their tiny capillary muscles have contracted to their maximum. They then return to the hot water tub and repeat the action. Many of these people claim that they were sick before they started this hot and cold treatment and that now they are cured. They all believe this procedure makes them so healthy they never get sick.

To me, this makes lots of sense. They are exercising their peripheral blood vessels and structures. They are also exercising the very important temperature regulating system of the human body. These people better tolerate the cold in winter and the heat in summer compared to others. I, myself, shower every morning starting with warm water, then make the water hot until I feel my muscles relax. Then suddenly, I turn the cold water all the way up and turn off the warm water. I let cold water hit my head first, then my back and then my chest until I no longer feel the coldness of the water.

When you first begin this exercise, the cold water seems almost intolerable, but as time goes on, you will find this one of the most refreshing feelings you can experience. Please start this exercise in summertime so the shock is not so great.

For those of you who suffer from icy hands and feet, please practice this exercise. This condition will improve and so will your blood pressure.

Chunging for Hypertension

High blood pressure is extremely dangerous, and you must consult your physician before you practice Chunging for Hypertension. I would like to warn those people who are now taking blood pressure medicine: you must *not* immediately stop taking your medicine when you begin Chunging for Hypertension. Some types of hypertension absolutely need medicine. But I believe that high blood pressure can be cured or at least controlled by the following:

1. Minimize salt intake and drink lots of water.

2. Stop all caffeine and nicotine intake.

3. Stop drinking carbonated beverages.

4. Avoid stress. Practice Parasympathetic Chunging, as outlined in the next chapter.

5. Exercise twice per week. Perspiring eliminates salt and other toxic wastes which cause hypertension.

6. Practice Breath Chunging, which will reduce stress. Directions are in the chapter on Breathing.

7. Practice Foot Chunging and thermo-regulating capillary exercise.

If you live by the guidelines mentioned above, 90% of the time you can cure essential hypertension (high blood pressure which has no definite cause) without the use of any medicine.

Control Stress Any Time

It has been proven that one of the major causes of human illness is stress. The main reason stress causes disease is that stress stimulates the sympathetic nervous system. When this system is stimulated, the nerve endings and the adrenal glands secrete epinephrine and norepinephrine, more commonly called adrenalin. These are essential, very important ingredients which cause the human body to respond properly to stressful situations by causing the heart to pump faster, elevating blood pressure, increasing the glucose content of the blood, and strengthening the skeletal muscles.

For a person involved in persistent and excessive stressful situations, these sympathetic effects induce diseases such as:

1. Heart disease, by making the heart work harder.

2. Hypertension, by constricting the blood vessels and increasing the power of heart contractions.

3. Indigestion, by diminishing intestinal movement and by reducing digestive enzyme production. This

decreases excretions from the salivary, gastric, and pancreatic glands and from the gall-bladder.

4. Allergic rhinitis, by drying up the surface of the nasal cavity.

5. Reddened eyes, by decreasing production of tears.

6. Difficulty in urination, by relaxing urinary bladder muscles and constricting the passageway of urine.

7. Premature ejaculation.

8. Elevated the blood sugar and cholesterol levels.

Physicians are well equipped to fight these problems by using pills for heart disease and hypertension, elixirs for indigestion, sprays for rhinitis, drops for red eyes, catheters for bladder retention, and so on.

Fortunately, a patient with these sympathetic nervous system problems does not have to rely only on these external sources for help. You can utilize internal natural help, the marvelous parasympathetic nervous system.

The Parasympathetic Nervous System

The human body has another nervous system called the parasympathetic nervous system which can counteract almost all sympathetic nervous system effects. These functions are almost always automatically in balance. The two systems together are called the autonomic nervous system.

When the sympathetic nervous system is over-stimulated by excessive and persistent stressful situations, human beings can activate the parasympathetic system by changing their behavior. Occasionally, the autonomic regulatory system needs help by deliberate stimulation of the parasympathetic nervous system.

People practice parasympathetic nervous system stimulation without knowing it. Here are a few examples:

1. Baseball players frequently chew gum when they are playing a tense game. Chewing gum enhances production of saliva. Secretion of saliva is an action of the parasympathetic system.

2. Many people eat when they are under stress. Eating promotes intestinal movement (peristalsis) and the secretion of digestive juices which are both effects of the parasympathetic nervous system.

3. A person under stress often cries, which relieves tension and red, itchy eyes. Tearing is another parasympathetic nervous system effect.

4. Some people blush when they are embarrassed or sexually aroused. Blushing is a parasympathetic function.

These acts, which promote salivary secretion, peristalsis, tearing, and blushing, stimulate the parasympathetic nervous system, counteracting the ill effects of the over-stimulated sympathetic nervous system. This is brought on by the secretion of acetylcholine at the parasympathetic nerve endings.

Normally, when the parasympathetic nervous system is stimulated, the following will happen as a result:

1. The heart will beat slower.

2. Blood pressure will be lowered by the decreasing force of heart contractions and will prevent a heart attack by dilating the coronary arteries.

3. Digestion of food will be aided by promoting intestinal movement and production and excretion of digestive juices.

4. Dryness in the nose and sinuses will disappear by the proper moistening of the nasal cavity.

5. Eye redness will disappear through the increased flow of tears.

6. Urination will become easier by strong contractions of the bladder muscles and by dilation of the urethra.

7. Parasympathetic stimulation helps the erection of the penis and delays ejaculation.

As you can see, all the normal parasympathetic effects are good for you. By Parasympathetic Chunging, we can eliminate many of the symptoms and signs of many common illnesses which are stress-related.

Parasympathetic Chunging should be the first approach to stress, rather than trying to solve these stress-induced problems by taking drugs.

Parasympathetic Chunging

In a stressful situation, rather than seeking medicine to calm your 'nerves', you should first try to calm yourself with these easy Parasympathetic Chunging Exercises.

1. Calming your mind is the key. Calming your mind makes your heart beat slower. Slowing down your heart's pumping rate is the most important and major function of the parasympathetic nervous system.

   When stress seems to be getting the better of you, you can calm your mind and body by performing the Breath Chunging exercises. You can do this anytime, anyplace. Breath Chunging increases peristalsis of the intestines, a function of the parasympathetic nervous system. Please do not misinterpret this advice to mean simple deep breathing. Breathing by using the chest wall, stimulates the sympathetic nervous system, which only produces *more* adrenalin. Read the chapter on Breath Chunging for proper breathing.

2. Try this tongue exercise. Rub your gums front to back with your tongue. This causes more saliva to flow, which also increases intestinal movement, increases production of digestive enzymes, and also neutralizes excess stomach acid which is produced by the stimulation of the sympathetic nervous system.

If you are involved in a stressful situation every day, practice regular meditation. The key to meditation is to calm your mind and do abdominal breathing.

One further parasympathetic stimulation which I recommend is that both men and women sleep without bottom underwear.

Sleeping without underwear enhances morning erections in men which are harder and last longer. This stimulates the production of acetylcholine continuously from the parasympathetic nerve endings. Sleeping without underwear also helps prevent scrotal varicose veins, which is one of the causes of male infertility. Keeping testicles in a cooler surrounding makes for better, normal, and production of more sperm. Testicles in a warmer surrounding make abnormal and fewer sperm. This is a medically proven fact.

Women sleeping without underwear will develop less moisture in the vagina which lessens the chance of vaginal infection.

Conventional Exercise Is Wrong

Many Americans engage in exercise to shape up their bodies, lose fat, and build muscle. Their goal is to make themselves look better, get stronger, and move faster. To achieve this goal, they push themselves hard, puffing and huffing until they are in a state of shortness of breath, with pain in the muscles and joints due to minor microscopic traumas. This type of exercise is very wrong.

When exercising, your cells need the following factors:

1. Sufficient nutrition.

2. Sufficient oxygen supply.

3. Proper elimination of waste products.

If these three requirements of exercise are not met, some damage will occur to the body. For instance, when a person has shortness of breath brought on by too strenuous exercise, his cells are suffering from a lack of oxygen. This is a very dangerous condition.

When deprived of oxygen, cells become sick. A body can sustain some dysfunctional cells, but the weakening of many cells puts an additional burden on the rest of the body.

Fortunately, before the age of forty, most cells can handle the toxic effects of a temporary lack of oxygen; even if some cells are damaged, they can be quickly repaired.

After the age of forty, cells cannot be replaced as quickly as when younger. This is why, in older people, exercise to the point of shortness of breath often leads to serious health problems.

If you see someone performing Chinese exercises, you will notice that all the movements are very slow, smooth, and coordinated with breathing. It is relaxed and graceful, more like slow dancing than like pure exercise. These exercises can be performed daily even by the oldest people. Many Americans feel that this isn't exercise at all because it is too 'easy'. On the contrary, slow Chunging exercise (like the Chinese exercise) serves its purpose well because it will keep you healthy and prevent disease.

For Americans, exercise is not exercise without shortness of breath and pain. "No pain, no gain" is often repeated in locker rooms and health clubs. We Americans never consider the true long term ill effects of exercise. What we consider to be ill effects are painful, debilitating infirmities such as tennis elbow, sprained ankles, and knee injuries. We only think about the damage to the body that we can see or feel.

When you are short of breath, your cells lack oxygen, which is called oxygen debt. Basically, you are suffocating your entire body on a cellular level. It takes two hours for your body to recover after each period of exhaustive exercise—you must not only supply your body with a normal amount of oxygen, but you literally have to repay each cell the oxygen debt.

You wouldn't want to suffocate yourself for even two minutes. Why would anyone suffocate their cells for two hours due to over-exhaustive exercise?

Occasionally, especially as we get older, it even takes several days to recover completely from over-exertion. The feeling of deep fatigue the day after exercise is the symptom that you have been doing the wrong type of exercise or that you have been working too hard.

If you are over the age of forty, you should not engage in 'exercise' which induces shortness of breath and exhaustion. When I see a middle aged man who is jogging or running in obvious pain, his face red from exertion, I pity him because I know he is doing more harm to his body than good. Although runners over forty may claim they feel good, they usually look older than their age, and many of them lose interest in sex.

Golf, like walking, is good exercise. It has been said that a golfer never wastes time when playing golf because he will extend his functional life by the same length of time that he spends playing. To me, this makes sense. No American golfer ever pushes himself to the point of shortness of breath during golf; his metabolism is not accelerated enough to produce dangerous free radicals, unless he becomes too emotionally involved. (Japanese golfers, on the other hand, do drive themselves unmercifully when playing the game.)

There are many other hidden, long-lasting injuries that can be induced by improper exercise.

Unforeseen problems can arise from continual and drastic over-exercise. For instance, most people think that body-builders are very healthy. This is not true. The goal of body building is hypertrophy of the muscles. Hypertrophy means excessive enlargement. This is an abnormal condition caused by overworking muscles.

To give you a better picture of the dangers of body building, let me compare it with hypertrophy of the heart muscle. The hearts of people suffering from prolonged hypertension become enlarged just like bodybuilders' muscles. The heart of a person with hypertension must pump his blood through narrowed arteries. This puts his heart under an inordinate amount of strain. As this condition is allowed to continue, the heart is continually over-exercised, trying to push blood through the clogged arteries. This hard workout induces heart muscle build-up; the heart becomes larger.

An enlarged heart needs more oxygen and nutrition, but the blood vessels supplying the heart cannot meet the heart's needs, causing the heart to become diseased. Eventually, it will lead to heart failure.

In the same way, when a bodybuilder places too much strain on any muscle, the muscle will become hypertrophic. Creating bigger muscles may mean stronger muscles in terms of weight lifting, but bigger muscles do not increase the body's strength in terms of general health. Bodybuilders unnecessarily enlarge the muscles which should remain small for normal functional life. Bodybuilders actually lose some of their range of motion due to the condition known as being 'muscle bound'. That is, they have excessively enlarged muscles which would work better if they were not enlarged.

Expansion of this group of normally small muscles could pinch blood vessels and nerves which supply more essential muscles. Furthermore, these unnecessarily expanded muscles may consume more nutrition and oxygen than if they weren't enlarged, thus suffocating other nearby muscles.

Another hidden danger of improper exercise is the production of metabolic errors called 'free radicals'. These dangerous chemical errors are a frequent result of exertion to the point of shortness of breath. Free radicals can be formed when there is not enough oxygen available for normal metabolism.

Free radicals are toxic products that attack other molecules indiscriminately. They float around in the body, doing various kinds of damage. They may randomly join with other chemicals to produce who knows what. They often produce chemical chain reactions, which change critically important enzymes or vital giant molecules such as DNA. Free radicals are a major cause of aging and cell damage.

Conventional exercise totally neglects the body-cleansing effect of exercise. A great many conventional exercises do not accomplish this valuable cleansing. Popular exercises concentrate on muscle use and development.

In contrast, all Chunging exercises are designed to gently clean the body on a cellular level, particularly when combined with Breath Chunging.

The point of many Chunging exercises is to increase the range of motion in the joints, and to maintain flexibility into old age. If enough gentle Chunging exercises are done to maintain joint flexibility, good muscle tone will also be maintained throughout your life.

If muscle tone *is* maintained, bone degeneration will not take place. That is, there will be little loss of bone mass due to aging.

None of these goals of Chunging exercises are beyond the reach of anyone, regardless of your physical condition or age. Fortunately, it is never too late to start improving your range of motion, muscle tone, and the condition of your bones. Chunging exercises can make you more flexible and more physically fit for the rest of your life.

The purpose of exercise is to make you healthy and disease-free and to allow the body to move over its entire range of motion. This is accomplished by:

1. Eliminating cellular waste.

2. Metabolizing excess nutrients.

Exercise makes you healthy by helping your cells eliminate excess nutrients and waste. Once a cell ingests nutrients, the nutrients have to be metabolized or stored as fat. The waste has to go out of the cell completely. If not excreted from the cell, the waste acts as a poison.

The cell, which previously had retained nutrients, begins collecting fat droplets in its cytoplasm. Unless you exercise, these fat droplets become larger and finally disturb the cell's normal function. Again, think about the theory of flow of *ki.* The energy that came into the cell must get out of the cell. If the *ki* (energy) gets stagnant, it will induce disease in the cell, especially in muscle cells. You need regular exercise of the whole body's muscles to clean out all the nutrients and waste, just like you have to move your bowels regularly.

The organs of the human body are mostly cleansed by blood. Blood brings in nutrition, and then takes away waste. But there are many parts of the human body which have little blood supply, like ligaments and some parts which have no blood supply, like cartilage. The most fibrous tissue of the human body has a lack of blood circulation. These tissues are dependent upon diffusion and osmosis for their exchange of nutrition and waste. However, this exchange is often not enough to keep these tissues healthy. They need compression and expansion to keep their cells clean.

For example, most joints are covered with cartilage, which has no blood supply. To maintain healthy joints, the whole surface of the joint must be gently compressed and expanded. This results in waste being squeezed out during compression, and an intake of nutrients during expansion. Most conventional exercises promote limited motion of joints. Running, for example, involves limited motion of the hip, knees, and feet—not the whole range of motion. Chunging Deep Knee Bending promotes a wider range of motion of hip joints, and a full range of motion of knee, ankle, and foot joints, without jarring the tender cartilage of the knee.

Retaining the whole range of motion in all the joints of the body is one of the keys to keeping your body young. Stiffer joints are older joints. Supple joints are Chunger joints. Use the Chunging exercises daily to keep flexible and fit.

Author's Note* I hope I am not discouraging people who are under forty from engaging in exhaustive exercise. If you are under forty, and in good health, the beneficial effects of pushing your body to the limit are greater than the harmful effects of shortness of breath.

Eyes, Ears and Nose

Most people who exercise believe they can improve only their heart or skeletal muscles. They are surprised to learn that there are other exercises besides cardiovascular exercises.

A common mistake of Western thought is to neglect the other organs of the body. Yes, proper cardiovascular exercise will make your heart Chunger, but other exercises will improve other organs as well. Typical exercises do not take into account organs such as the brain, eyes, nose, and ears. Proper exercise should include all of these neglected organs. You *can* improve your eyes, nose, and ears. Proper exercise should be a whole-body experience.

People accept without question that eyesight worsens with age. They simply get glasses or contact lenses. As more time passes, their eyes continue to become worse. They may even develop cataracts or other conditions which require surgery. Hearing loss, too, is accepted as inevitable, and some problems probably can't be avoided. But it is not inevitable. Many people retain excellent hearing all their life.

I am convinced that there are easy ways to prevent these problems: do these Chunging exercises for your eyes and ears every day.

Cleansing Exercises for the Eyes

As a person ages, the most common eye problems that occur are nearsightedness or farsightedness. These problems are caused by a weakening of the focusing power of the lens and eyeball. The inability to focus properly develops mainly because the muscles around the eye are not properly exercised.

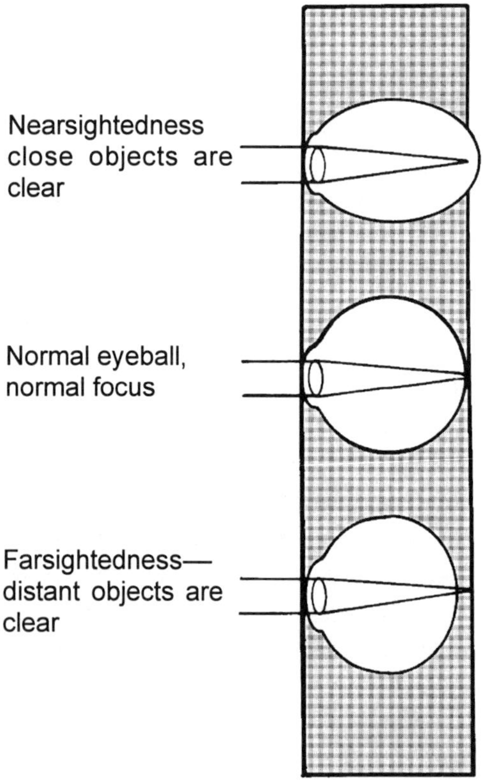

Consider, for example, the child who spends all day watching TV and reading books. He surely has a greater chance of becoming nearsighted than a child who spends all his time on outdoor activities, which would cause his eyes to constantly refocus on objects at various distances away from him.

As you can see in this picture, the eye is surrounded by seven muscles located between the eyeball and its bony socket.

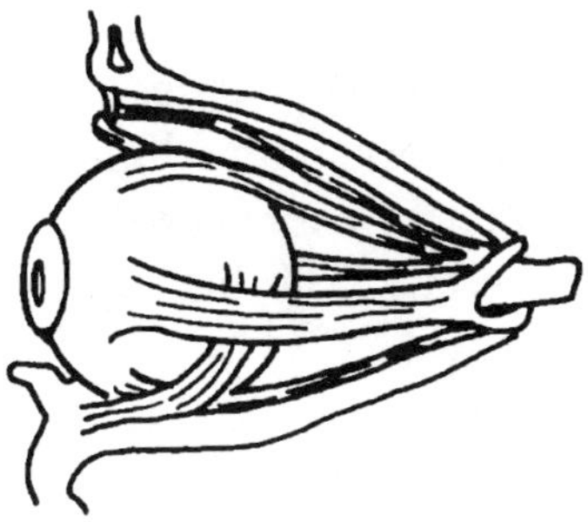

If these muscles are not properly exercised, they will deteriorate, and fat will accumulate around the muscle, just as happens in any skeletal muscle.

The dual effect of deterioration of the muscles and uneven fat accumulation around the eyeball will change the shape of the eyeball which will adversely affect eyesight. In order to avoid this, you must properly exercise the muscles of the eye.

Cataracts form when abnormal chemicals cloud the lens, causing the lens to become opaque. If we were able to prevent the collection of these chemicals on the lens, cataracts would not develop. Stimulating the production of tears and helping the circulation of blood to the eyes will promote healthier eyes.

One must simply assist the natural washing process in order to prevent the development of cataracts. The following Eye Chunging exercises are cleansing exercises for the eyes.

This exercise will keep your eyeballs in optimum shape by strengthening eye muscles and eliminating accumulated fat .

Step 1. Rub your hands together until your fingers get warm.

Step 2. Close your eyes. Then place your fingers over your eyes and press lightly until you can feel the movement of your eyeballs. The warmth and pressure generated by your hands promotes better circulation to your eyes.

Step 3. Inhale a full breath through your nose. As you hold your breath, turn your eyes from center to far right three times and back to the center before you exhale slowly through your mouth

Step 4. Using the same procedure as in step three, turn your eyes from looking straight forward to the far left. On each movement of these exercises, you should move your eyes far enough that you can feel the muscles working.

Step 5. Using the same breathing pattern, move your eyeballs from the center position to as far up as you can, then back to the normal position. Remember the point of proper breathing is to give your cells extra oxygen.

Step 6. Using the same breathing pattern, move your eyeballs from the center until you are looking down as far as possible. (Repeat all the Eye Chunging steps at least three times.)

Eye Chunging Under Water

Do this exercise when your face is clean and any make-up has been removed. Eye make-up especially must be gently and carefully removed before Eye Chunging Under Water.

Step 1. Fill a clean pan or bowl with lukewarm water. As this tends to get the front of your hair wet, you can use two coffee cups, one for each eye.

Step 2. Inhale deeply through your nose, then holding your breath, place your face into the water leaving the eyes open.

Step 3. Repeat Eye Chunging Under Water one to three times, for the length of time you are holding each breath.

The surface of the eye is constantly cleansed with tears. These tears originate in the lacrimal glands and flow down through

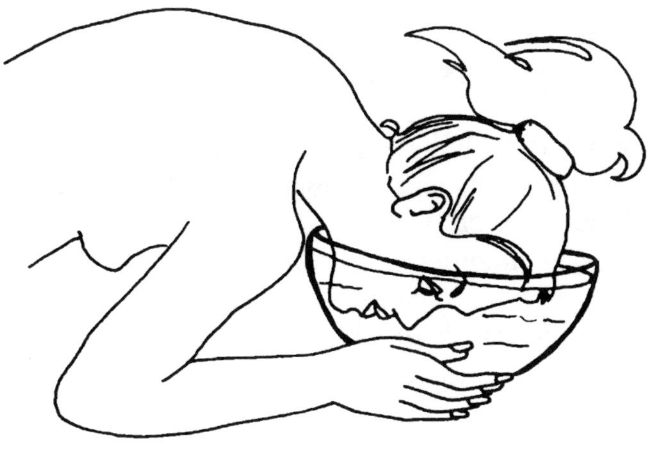

the lacrimal ducts into the nasal cavity. Water helps stimulate the production of tears without any harmful effects. Water also helps to clean the surface of the eye.

Pollutants are everywhere in the air nowadays. You must do these cleansing exercises daily. Those in any occupation where there is pollen, chemicals, or dust have great need to make these exercises part of their daily lives. Eye Chunging Under Water is also especially beneficial to people who frequently use computers; computer users often stare at the screen so absorbed in their project that they forget to blink their eyes often enough, and they go long periods without changing their point of focus.

It has been written by some Taoist therapists that this exercise can prevent and even improve existing cataracts. This exercise is particularly helpful to those people suffering from itchy eyes due to allergies.

After you start cleaning your eyes, you may notice a little redness around the eyes and possibly some eye discharge. This will disappear within a month if you continue to clean your eyes. After a few years of Eye Chunging, you will notice improvement in your eyesight.

Author's Note* My wife and I practice these exercises daily because we understand the logic behind them. Since we started these exercises, both of us are sure that our eyesight has noticeably improved. However, I can offer no proof from my personal experience that can substantiate the claims of these Taoists that these exercises can improve or prevent cataracts.

Cleansing Exercises for the Ears

After the age of forty, many people notice that their hearing becomes worse. Also, they begin to hear occasional, high-pitched, annoying sounds.

Sound waves hit the eardrum, causing the eardrum to vibrate. These vibrations are then transmitted to the inner ear by three little ear bones, each of which is connected in turn to the other by tiny joints.

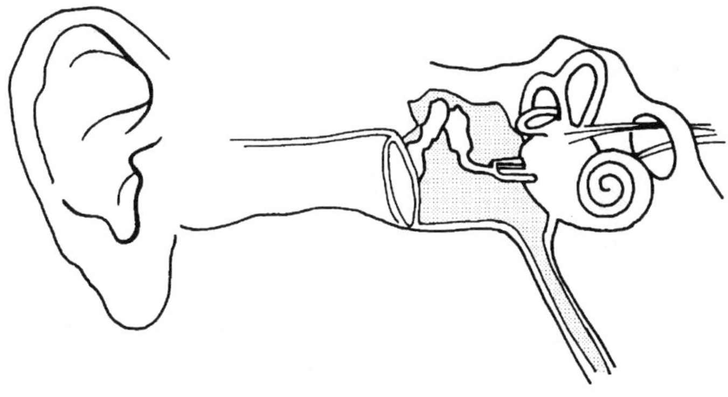

It is my opinion that the major causes of hearing loss due to aging are the loss of elasticity of the eardrum, stiffening of the ear bones' tiny joints, weakening of the muscles surrounding the ear bones, and accumulation of waste in the inner ear. The following exercises are designed to strengthen these small muscles and keep the delicate small joints mobile.

Ear Chunging by Popping

Put your index fingers in both ears firmly as though you were trying to block out sound. Then remove your index fingers quickly. You will hear a popping sound. Repeat this procedure three times per day.

This exercise will cause your eardrums to vibrate, helping them to keep their elasticity.

Ear Chunging by Popping will force the joints of your little ear bones to move over their entire range, preventing stiffening of the tiny joints and preventing weakening of the middle ear structure.

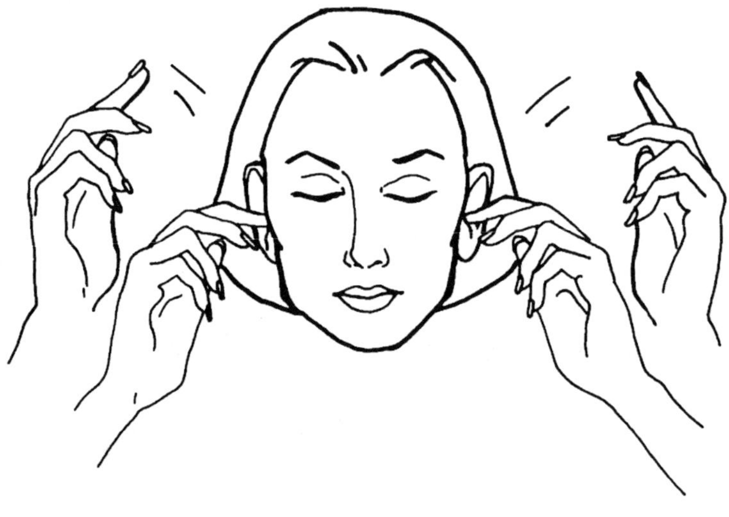

Ear Chunging by Snapping

With your palms on a table, place your index finger over your middle finger, and with a snapping motion, hit the table with your index finger.

Using this same type of motion, fold the back of your earlobe over with your middle finger and snap your index finger onto the mastoid bone. The mastoid is the lump you feel at the base of your skull right behind your ear.

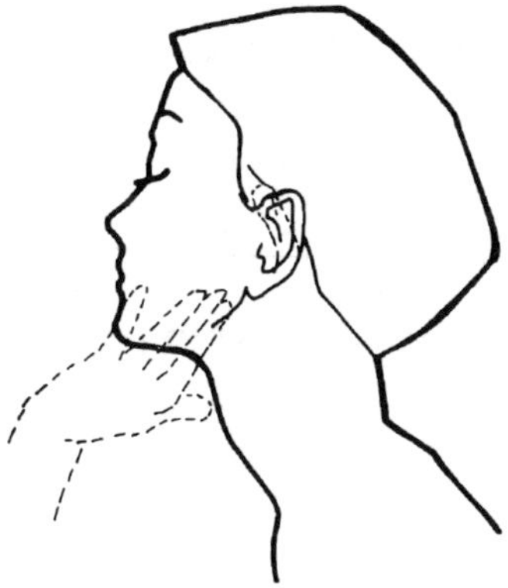

Snapping or tapping the mastoid bone just behind the ear agitates the inner ear which will help activate aging cells and help clear away abnormal accumulation of cellular waste. Repeat this exercise three times a day.

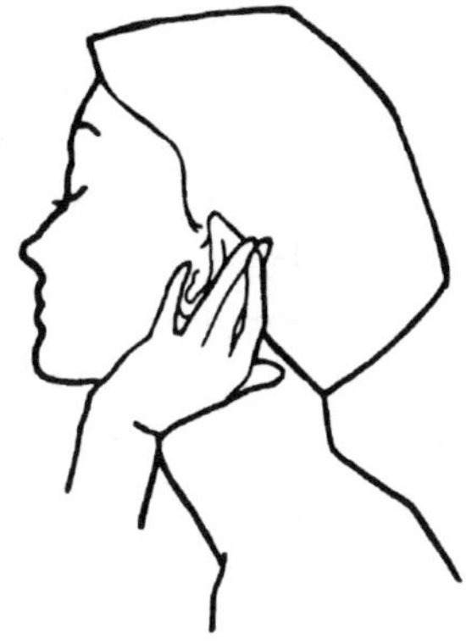

The inner ear contains organs which provide you with hearing and govern your sense of balance.

Ear Chunging also prevents or improves conditions which involve the sense of balance, such as vertigo.

Ear Chunging by Warming

Place your palms over your ears and rub your ears firmly until both ears feel warm. This will help circulation to your ears.

These ear exercises should be done in conjunction with the nasal cleansing exercises because your nasal cavities are connected to the ears by the Eustachian channels. In fact, many ear diseases originate from nasal infections.

I discussed these techniques with an ear specialist and he assured me that the degree of stimulation these exercises apply to the ear could not cause any damage.

These are gentle exercises. Needless to say, should you feel pain from eye or ear Chunging, you should discontinue the exercises and see your physician immediately.

Allergic Rhinitis and Sinusitis

Vicky H. is a seventeen year-old high school senior who suffered from chronic sinusitis. She constantly had a stuffy nose and had yellow, puss-like drainage. She had a swollen, achy face and frequent headaches and snored when she slept. She had none of these problems until the age of fifteen when she started showing signs of an allergy to pollen and dust. She went to a physician who prescribed antihistamines to be taken by mouth and also nasal sprays. At first these medicines seemed to help, but as the months went by, her allergy became worse and worse until, finally, she felt stuffy all the time.

Pollen and dust travel through the air into our upper respiratory tracts. However, the nose's interior surface, called the nasal mucosa, traps pollen or dust before it reaches the lungs. This membrane secretes small amounts of sticky mucous to trap or wash away the harmful pollen and dust.

For some reason, Vicky developed an extra sensitivity to pollen and dust so that her nasal mucosa produced a larger amount of mucous, causing her runny nose.

A runny nose is a self-protective mechanism to eliminate the harmful material. Antihistamines inhibit the production of mucous by the nasal mucosa, allowing the pollen and dust to accumulate instead of being carried away by mucous. This accumulation causes inflammation and infection which later becomes sinusitis.

While on vacation in Florida, Vicky swam in the pool every day. Gradually, she realized that her nose was clearing up. Her headaches disappeared, and by the time the vacation ended, Vicky thought she was over her problem. Even the snoring had stopped. When Vicky swam frequently, water traveled in and out of her nose. This water action helped wash away the harmful pollen and dust from her nasal cavities, causing her symptoms to disappear.

However, she did not have to go on vacation to eliminate her problem. The way to fight many airborne allergies is to rinse the interior of the nose. Vicky could have simply washed her nose at home by using the Nose Chunging techniques which I will describe on the next page. This solution is so simple—and so logical—I am always surprised when my patients tell me they never heard of such a thing.

Nose Chunging

This exercise is especially helpful if performed both in the morning and night.

> Step 1. Hold some water in both hands. Place your nose into the water and sniff in the water until you feel the water reach the top of the inside of your nose. (Stop before you start feeling pain.) Then let the water run out your nostrils. Repeat this five times, then blow your nose.
>
> Step 2. After you blow your nose, hold some water in one hand. Place your nose into the water and sniff in a nose-full. Then lean your head backwards gently, allowing the water in the nose to run down your throat. Swallow. Repeat three times.

After using this method for awhile, people suffering from allergies, sinusitis, or snoring may experience a large quantity of watery, post-nasal drip. This is a sign that the disease is disappearing. If you were to continue using this cleansing method, the extensive drainage would soon disappear, signaling the cure of the disease. Most patients start to feel better after three days using this method. In three weeks, they are usually cured.

If you live in a dry house or dry climate, your nose will feel wonderful, after the very first time you try Nose Chunging. I recommend that you continue this exercise as a preventative measure, no matter the humidity or season of the year.

The cleansing exercises I have introduced eliminate the cause of disease, not just the symptoms. Similarly, you should not suppress the normal functioning of the nasal mucosa with medicine unless absolutely necessary. If you are experiencing acute discomfort and distress due to a severe allergy or infection, you must use medicine which your doctor prescribes while continuing to practice this cleansing exercise. It's always good to try to minimize the use of medicine.

Author's Note* A friend of mine, an ear, nose, and throat specialist, told me that he would recommend using normal saline solution (diluted salt water) instead of tap water. My wife and I have been using tap water and we have found that very satisfactory, but some people may be more comfortable using normal saline solution.

Ear Discomfort while Flying

There are many people who are afraid of traveling in airplanes because they experience severe ear aches due to sharp altitude changes. These ear aches are caused by the development of a difference between the pressure of the atmosphere and the pressure in the middle ear. People who have healthy noses and middle ears only experience tolerable discomfort while people who have inflammations or infections in their nasal cavities or middle ears often suffer extreme discomfort.

There are many pilots and flight attendants who must quit their jobs due to this intolerable pain. They were advised to practice Valsalva's maneuver, an unnatural way of increasing the pressure in the nasal cavities that will forcibly open the channel between the nose and middle ear. To perform this maneuver, hold your nose shut, close your mouth and blow. Although this often clears the ears, I consider Valsalva's maneuver dangerous as it can easily introduce germs from the nasal cavity into the middle ear, causing ear infections.

I used to suffer from severe ear aches when traveling by air. However, since I began practicing Nose Chunging, I have not experienced any severe ear problems when flying. I have advised many of my patients and friends with similar problems, and they all have benefited from my instructions.

Remember, the nose is connected with both the ears and eyes. If you have a healthy nose, Nose Chunging will prevent diseases of both the eyes and ears.

Snoring

Snoring develops when you have abnormal nasal passages. The cause of this may be sinusitis or allergic rhinitis or simply a dry nose. I strongly recommend that a person who snores use these cleansing exercises. Many snorers who wash their nasal cavities with water find their nasal passages open, thus freeing them from the snoring problem.

The Head and Neck

One of the first visible places to show signs of aging is the skin of the neck. As people grow older, large wrinkles and folds begin to appear. If you follow my instructions, many of these wrinkles will disappear, or at least, existing wrinkles will not become worse.

Many people think that wrinkles develop because the skin loses its elasticity with aging. This is true. However, loss of elasticity is only half of the problem. The other half, which is usually neglected, is the loss of musculature under the skin.

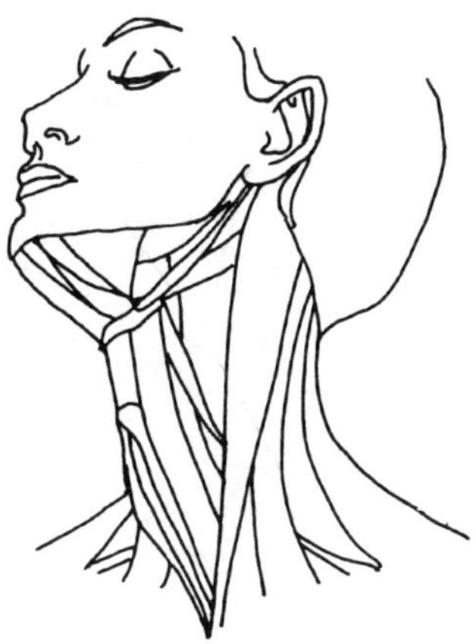

A person who has strong, well-developed stomach muscles, appears to have healthy, firm stomach skin. In the same way, a person who has strong, healthy facial muscles will appear to have healthy, young, facial skin.

Wrinkles under the chin and neck are due to the weakening and loss of muscle tone of a superficial neck muscle called the platysma (which is pronounced *pla tis' ma*). Chin Chunging exercises will develop this muscle and will prevent and even eliminate existing wrinkles in this area.

Chin Chunging

To keep the platysma and the muscles around your mouth firm and to improve a double chin:

Step 1. Exhale through the mouth.

Step 2. Inhale through the nose. While inhaling, smile an open-mouthed smile with teeth clenched and contract the jaw and neck muscles as tight as you can. Hold it until you are finished inhaling.

Step 3. Exhale through the mouth again. Repeat this exercise at least five times.

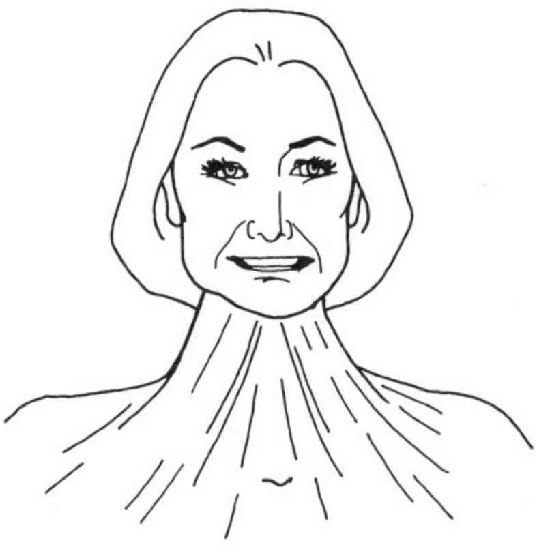

Notice how many different muscles are affected by this exercise; the tension pulls the muscles of the upper chest as well as the neck and jaw muscles. By toning the platysma, fat deposits are reduced and therefore wrinkles are minimized.

Cheek Chunging

This exercise has been used in the Orient for thousands of years to promote better health and a youthful appearance.

> Step 1. Insert tongue between your upper lip and teeth. Sweep your tongue from right to left. Then sweep from left to right. Repeat twice.
>
> Step 2. Insert tongue between your lower lip and teeth. Sweep your tongue from right to left. Then sweep from left to right. Repeat twice.
>
> Step 3. With tongue in the same position as in steps one and two, rotate your tongue around your whole mouth (upper and lower) from right to left. Then rotate from left to right. Repeat twice. By this time you will notice that saliva is gathering on the floor of your mouth, and your tongue may be tired. Swallow the saliva and repeat exercise.

Cheek Chunging has also been used for indigestion and abdominal pain as well as for many allergic disorders and gum disease. These claims are logical since this exercise eliminates allergens and food particles that collect in the mouth. It promotes circulation to the gums, and helps digestion by producing more saliva. Saliva is a basic solution which can neutralize and dilute excess acid in the stomach, and it also contains enzymes which aid in digestion.

Remember this exercise when you have heartburn and you are far away from the antacids in your medicine cabinet.

Eliminating Face Wrinkles

One of the contributing factors in the development of skin wrinkles is poor circulation. The layer between the skin and the underlying muscles contains blood vessels. The following exercise is designed to make these blood vessels stronger and healthier.

> Step 1. Place palms on both sides of the face firmly. Rub up and down vigorously, not to create friction between the skin of the face and the hands, but to cause the underlying muscles to move against your facial bones.
>
> Step 2. Using same procedure in Step 1, rub entire scalp.

This exercise will also help eliminate headaches. Many headaches occur as a result of abnormal dilation or constriction of this layer of blood vessels.

Eliminating Wrinkles around the Eyes

Practicing the exercises found in the chapter on Eyes, Ears and Nose, will eliminate wrinkles and bags under the eyes.

So-called bags under the eyes are really fat deposits and the occasional retention of water in the tissue of the eye lids. The eye exercises will eliminate wrinkles by diminishing the collection of fat and water around the rest of the eye and by toning the facial muscles.

Prevent and Cure Headaches

Many people suffer from frequent headaches while others have never had a headache in their entire lives. The major cause of headaches is the accumulation of abnormal chemicals in the brain.

The brain is composed of trillions of nerve cells and the cells of supporting structures. These cells are working all the time, and therefore, producing waste constantly. The only way to minimize these waste products is to drink water, breathe properly, and ingest fewer toxic food additives.

When you take medicine to relieve a headache, you are only counteracting the pain. This does not eliminate the waste products of the brain cells which are the cause of the headache. To better understand this, I would like to introduce the case of Annie G.

Annie G. is now 42 years old. She is a working mother who has two children. At the age of 35, she was experiencing occasional, mild headaches. She took aspirin or acetaminophen which made her headaches better. The headaches kept recurring and getting worse. She visited her family physician, who told her the headaches were caused by stress and tension from her busy schedule and responsibilities. He prescribed a stronger pill that stopped her headaches better than over-the-counter medicine. After a time, however, her headaches got worse and were radiating to the front of her head, and sometime were so severe she couldn't work. The headaches were often associated with nausea. She was referred to a neurologist who found nothing wrong on physical examination but conducted a number of expensive tests to rule out any possible brain tumor or other organic disease. All the findings of the tests were normal. The neurologist then gave her another newly developed headache pill and referred her to me as a gynecologist since her headaches were accentuated before each menstrual period.

When I saw Annie G. two years ago, she was an intellectual, slightly overweight lady who appeared tired. The physical examination was normal except her blood pressure which was slightly higher than usual. During the interview, Annie G. told me she moves her bowels once every third to fifth day. I find that constipation is often an important factor in headaches. She was frequently eating out and consuming large quantities of soda and salt (salt is a major cause of hypertension and headaches). She said she can't find time to spend in the bathroom or for cooking at home. She also tells me she hates the taste of water, so I knew she doesn't drink enough water.

After this physical exam and interview, I explained to Annie G. the importance of daily bowel movements and drinking large quantities of water, and also the possible harmful effects of soda and salty food. Annie G. understood well and she started drinking six glasses of water a day and moving her bowels daily by practicing gastro-intestinal Chunging. She also stopped drinking soda and minimized her salt intake.

Three months later she had no more severe headaches and missed no more work. Annie is now forty-four and a lot happier. Her blood pressure is normal. She feels healthier than two years ago and exercises more simply because she feels better now. In fact, she *is* Chunger than she was two years earlier. She has been free of headaches, for a whole year.

Most headaches are caused by either abnormal chemicals or from the build-up of normal chemicals in the human body. Giving drugs to Annie G. merely counteracted the action of the headache-causing chemicals; it did not eliminate the cause. The bad chemicals were retained in her body, their concentration getting higher, and the symptoms of headache getting worse. Following my Chunging exercises, Annie minimized absorption of the headache-causing chemicals by daily bowel movements and diluted the chemicals by drinking water which also flushed the chemicals from her body

Chunging Exercises for Headaches

Headaches may also be induced by spasms of the neck and facial muscles and abnormal dilation and constriction of blood vessels of the head.

Step 1. Practice Chin and Cheek Chunging described earlier in this chapter. This will improve circulation to the head by correcting any abnormal dilation and constriction of blood vessels.

Step 2. Practice Chin and Neck Chunging. These exercises will relieve muscle spasms of the neck and face, thereby eliminating headaches of this type.

Step 3. Practice the cleansing exercises for the nose, eyes, and ears, since some headaches are related to the diseased condition of these organs.

Step 4. Practice the Figure-eight Exercise for Headaches described on the following page.

Figure-eight Exercise for Headaches

1. Make a fist of your right hand and press the area between your eye and your ear firmly with the knuckle of your thumb.

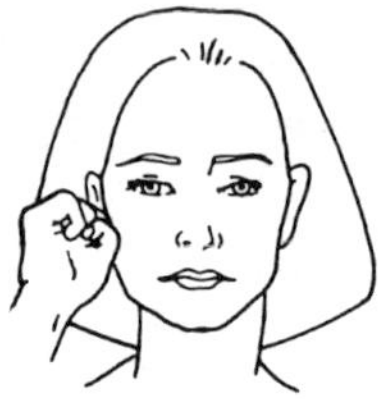

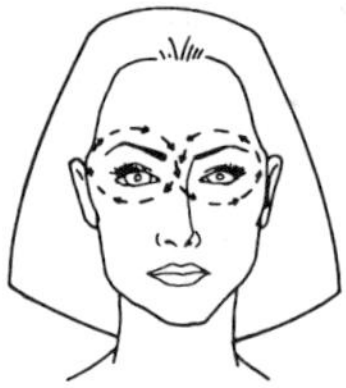

2. Make a figure-eight around both eyes, returning knuckles to the same position.

3. Make a figure-eight around your ear and face, across your chin to the starting position.

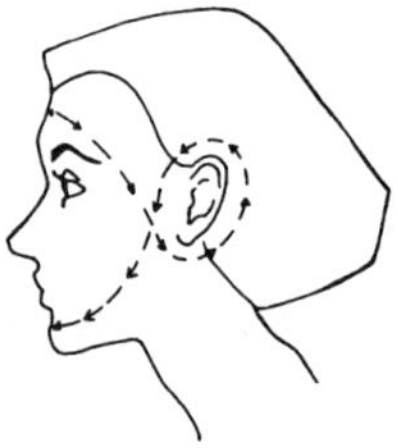

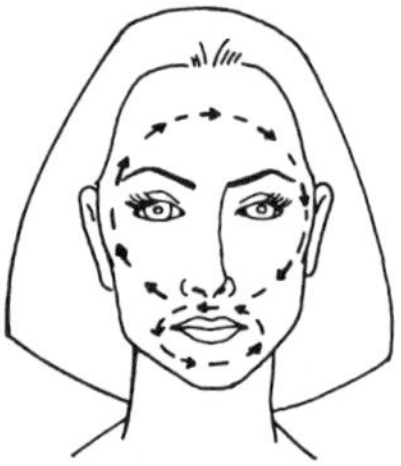

4. Make a figure-eight around your face and mouth.

5. Using the left hand, make a fist and repeat these exercises with the knuckle of the left hand.

Do these exercises when you have a headache and you will immediately feel a lessening in the intensity of the headache.

Author's Note* If you follow all the advice I have given in this section and still experience frequent headaches, you should see a neurologist since your headaches could be related to an organic disease.

Spine Chunging

Spine Chunging is the way you can make your appearance younger looking and your movements Chunger.

To appear younger, you must have good posture and maintain good proportion in your body. This is only possible by keeping your spine healthy and by eliminating the excess deposits of fat around the abdomen and hips.

To move like a younger person, you must have supple joints, especially the joints of the spine. You may remember the walk of Marilyn Monroe. On each step she took, her whole body moved, flexing and extending the joints of the spine, hip, knee, ankle, shoulder, wrist, etc. If you can imitate the walk of 'MM', you are indeed a young person, no matter what your age is.

Spine Chunging will improve your gait. As you get older, your pace tends to becomes slower because your steps become shorter. These exercises will loosen your joints and give you a new sense of confidence. You will take longer, more confident steps when walking.

The most important joints in the body are the joints of the spine. Besides your head, your entire body is governed through your spine. "A healthy spine means a healthy body," is the original philosophy of chiropractors and osteopaths. I cannot condemn a practitioner who claims he can cure many diseases by simply manipulating the spine, because every organ below the head is controlled by the nerves which travel down the spine.

The frame of the spine is composed of bones (vertebrae) and intervertebral discs. This frame encloses and protects the bundle of nerves which makes up the spinal cord.

This trunk of nerves is surrounded by a clear, thin liquid called spinal fluid, which extends for the length of the spine and into the brain. When a person fractures his skull, often one of the symptoms is that a clear liquid comes out of the ear. This is spinal fluid. It is a sign that the person is seriously injured and needs experienced medical help.

Between the vertebrae, there are holes called intervertebral foramen (*fo ra' men*). The roots of the nerves leave the spinal column and extend to their destinations through these holes.

Spinal injuries can cause pain or paralysis in any part of the body, depending on the location of the injury. By maintaining the muscles of the back through gentle Chunging exercises, you can do a great deal to prevent unnecessary spinal injuries. Sometimes, stepping on a pebble while walking down a sidewalk can put tremendous sideways stress on the back and spine. If the muscles are strong and the backbone flexible, it may hurt a lot, but may cause no real damage.

The Aging Spine

Over 90% of the population over the age of forty develops minor or major lower back problems. The evidence of an aging spine is:

1. Loss of elasticity of the discs.

2. Weakened vertebral bone.

3. Loss of muscular mass and strength around the spine and abdomen.

To Keep Your Spine Healthy

First, you must retain elasticity in the discs. Elasticity is lost when waste material builds up in the discs. Since circulation is poor around the discs, how do you eliminate waste? You simply compress and stretch your discs through bending, which squeezes out waste, and stretching, which sucks in the fresh nutrients. When you bend forward, you are compressing the front portion of your discs and at the same time, stretching the back portion.

Second, you must keep the bone mass of vertebrae strong by means of a weight-bearing exercise which has been proven to maintain good bone texture and prevent bone loss.

Third, you must maintain strong, healthy muscle around the spine and abdominal wall. These muscles support the spine and protect the vertebrae and discs from injury.

Spine Chunging is able to fulfill these needs and will prevent aging of the spine and also rejuvenate the spine if it has already aged.

How to Recognize Whether You Have an Aged Spine

A 'pot belly' or 'love handles' are a sign of an aged spine. It is proof of a loss of muscle mass and muscle strength around the spine and abdomen.

A person who has a stiff and aching back on awakening has an aging spine. This is a sign of loss of elasticity in the discs.

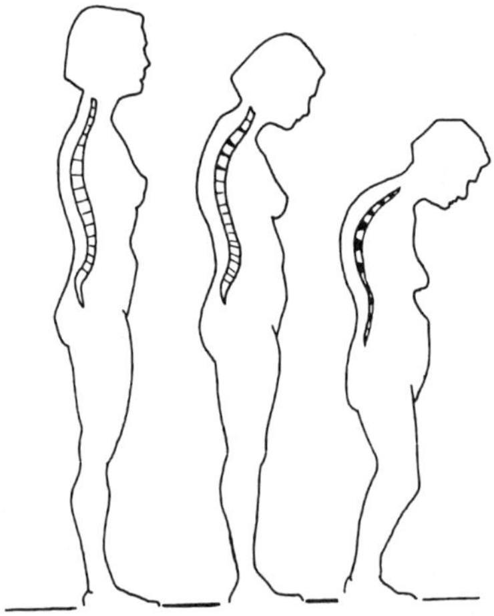

Even if you have no excess or abnormal curvature, you have an aging spine if you need a pillow to sleep. A person who has a young spine sleeps comfortably without a pillow. This is proof that that person has healthy lungs and a healthy heart.

There is a Korean saying, " higher pillows, sooner death." This is logical because people who have heart or lung problems can only sleep when their pillows are 'high'. They need a lot of neck support, either to prevent discomfort in their neck and back or to help them breathe more easily.

When you have practiced the Spine Chunging exercises for some time, you will notice, that, as your physical condition improves, you will need fewer or no pillows to sleep, meaning that your heart, lungs, and spine will be healthier than before. People who exercise even fifteen minutes a day will notice an improvement in posture.

The Most Important Exercise

Many people think walking is the most fundamental exercise. It is not. The most fundamental exercise is to sit up from a supine position. As you know, this is the first big step (after learning to roll over) that an infant conquers in his or her physical development.

Doing sit-ups is the only exercise which is able to eliminate a pot belly and love handles, as well as improve a stiff back and bad posture.

Long before the back problems arise, most people develop pot bellies. Even if a person were twenty and had a pot belly, his body would look older than a thirty-year-old who has no pot belly. This means that the twenty-year-old would not only look older, but actually be closer to death from disease and would not be as physically functional as the person who has lived ten years longer. This is a little-known fact of life.

The pot belly is a sign of aging in the spine. When you eliminate your pot belly and develop your abdominal muscles, you will make your spine young again.

At any age and condition, you can improve your spine and start eliminating your pot belly in only a few months.

Chunging Sit-ups

No one likes to do sit-ups. *Do them anyway.* If you truly want to remain physically functional into old age, do these sit-ups regularly:

> Step 1. Lie on your back. Bend your knees and latch your feet under something heavy to keep your feet on the ground. Support the back of your head with both hands.
>
> Step 2. Start exhaling through the mouth while pulling your upper body towards your knees. Finish exhaling.
>
> Step 3. Close your mouth. Slowly return to the supine position. You will notice that you will be automatically inhaling through your nose. Return to step one.

The sit-up exercise is the best exercise for your spine because it bends and extends your spine. Also, sit-ups develop the supporting muscles around the spine. If the muscles become weak, too much strain is placed on the bones and ligaments. Thus, building the muscles protects the spine from injuries. Sit-ups also build the abdominal muscles, which balance your weight distribution, further protecting the spine from injuries.

Many of you are unable to do even one single sit-up. Don't worry. Try to do the second most important exercise first.

Deep Knee Chunging

The second most important exercise is deep knee bending. I have described the Chunging technique for this old exercise in the chapter on Adult Diabetes. No one likes to do these exercises, either, unless they are in good shape to start with.

But the very ones who hate to do them or who can't do a deep knee bend at all are the people who need this exercise the most. There are many people who might be able to get into a squatting position, but are unable to get up again.

I strongly believe that this is an essential exercise for retaining a healthy body. Deep knee bends should be done every day. Stop bending at the waist when you have to pick something up from the floor. Make your leg muscles work. They *will* work—better and better each time you do it.

Like all Chunging exercises, deep knee Chunging should be done slowly and smoothly.

If you can feel tight muscles pulling—good. It just proves how much you need to use those exact muscles. They will improve in a few days. Just don't do so many knee bends the first day that you are too sore the next day and give up on knee bends altogether. Increase by one a day, or one every other day, if that is too fast. It took you a long time to get out of shape—don't be in too much of a rush to gain that strength back.

Arm and Back Chunging

This exercise is especially good for shoulder and upper back pain, and for prevention of pain from sedentary office jobs like word processing.

Step 1. Stand with your feet at shoulder width. Stretch your arms straight forward. Open both palms in front of your face. Reaching under your left hand, grasp below your left thumb with the fingers of the right hand.

Step 2. Press the back of your left hand with your right thumb. While exhaling through your mouth, extend your arms. At the same time, bend over as far as you can with your knees straight.

Step 3. Slowly inhale, while returning to the original position described in Step 1.

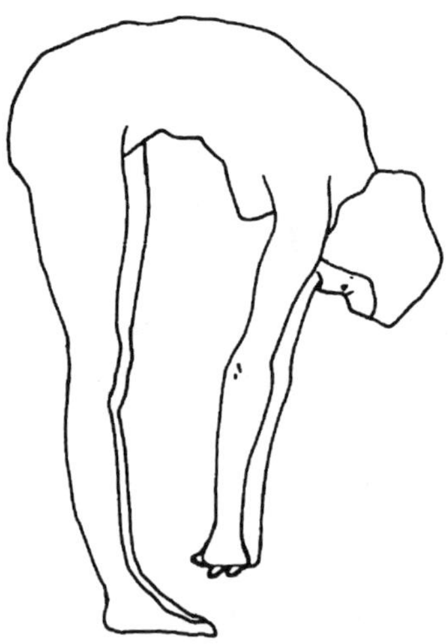

Step 4. Change hand positions. Repeat Steps 1-3.

This exercise may be combined with Shoulder Chunging, which is described on the following page.

Shoulder Chunging

This is the exercise which will prevent and cure frozen shoulders, as well as keep shoulder blades mobile.

Step 1. Clasp your hands together, interlocking your fingers.

Step 2. Exhale slowly through your mouth. Extend your arms so that both palms face the ceiling. Stare at the backs of your hands until you finish exhaling.

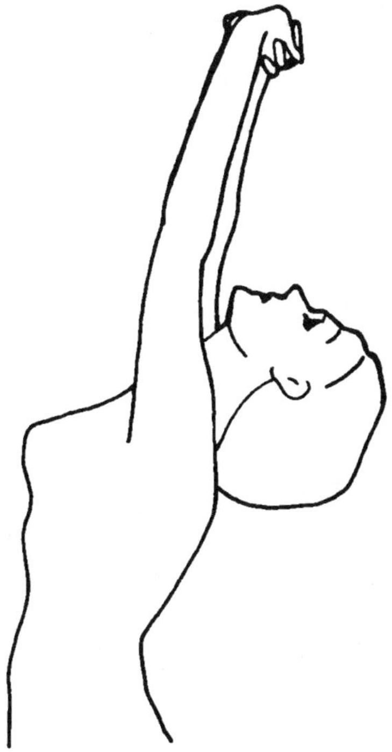

Step 3. Inhale through your nose and return to the original position.

Step 4. Exhale through your mouth as you bend, extending your arms so that your palms face the ground. Stare at the back of your hands until you finish exhaling.

Step 5. Inhale through your nose and return to the original position. Repeat this exercise five times.

Neck Chunging

To prevent a stiff neck, you must do this exercise whenever you have a few minutes. It can be done anytime.

Step 1. Start exhaling through your mouth as you lift your head back until your chin is pointing towards the ceiling. Keep looking upward towards your eyebrows until you are finished exhaling. Close your mouth. Return your head to its down position.

Step 2. Inhale through your nose while you bend your head down until your chin touches the upper part of your chest wall. Look sharply downwards towards your chin.

Step 3. Inhale through your nose. Begin exhaling through your mouth while you turn your head to the right. Stare to the right as far as you can. Start inhaling and return your head to its resting position. Repeat procedure while turning your head to the left.

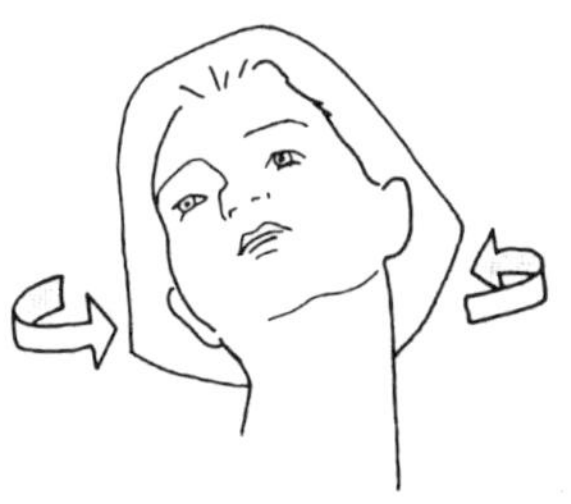

Step 4. Inhale though your nose and bend your head so that your chin rests on the upper part of your chest wall. Start exhaling through your mouth while rotating your head from right to left. Return to resting position. Inhale and repeat procedure, left to right.

You may hear a cracking or creaking sound. Do not worry; as long as you move slowly and stop before you turn so far that it hurts, you will not be harmed.

Repeat this exercise as often as you can. It will tone and strengthen the platysma muscle, eliminating excess fat deposits and thereby decreasing wrinkles. This exercise will also strengthen other neck muscles and increase the mobility of the cervical spine.

Chunging Push-ups

One of the fundamental physical activities is pushing objects. Maintaining this ability is very important for daily activity. This exercise strengthens your entire spine. I'm certain that all of you know how to do pushups. Remember to keep your entire body straight. The only new aspect that you must include is coordination of the exercise motions with your breathing.

Exhale when you stretch your arms. Inhale as you you bend your arms.

Because you are inhaling when your nose is close to the floor, make certain that you are not breathing in dust. Unless a floor is very clean, place a clean surface under your face, such as a sheet of plastic or even a book. This is one of the benefits of exercise mats; they keep your face off the floor. Even carpet which has just been vacuumed still contains dust, mites and microscopic bits of fiber, things you definitely don't want to inhale into your lungs.

Chin-up Chunging

Considering that human beings are descendants of the apes, the ability to hold your body's weight with your hands and arms should be natural. By retaining this ability, you can prevent many ailments and unnecessary joint pains of the whole body. This is a good exercise for stretching the spine's discs and muscles to their maximum extension. These movements open the vertebral foramen, releasing the nerve roots from compression.

- Chin-ups must be practiced as slowly as possible.
- Coordinate this exercise with breathing. Exhale when pulling up, inhale when going down.

The Essence of Chunging Exercises

The very essence of Chunging Exercises is wrapped up in three things:

1. Chunging exercises must be coordinated with Chunging breathing. This gets rid of more waste from the body through elimination of more carbon dioxide.

2. Chunging exercises must be those fundamental body movements which humans use for daily life.

3. Chunging exercises must use the full range of motion of the joint by stretching the muscle as far as it can go without pain.

Furthermore, any jarring of the joint or quick or fast movement are not Chunging exercises.

Why is this difference between conventional exercise and Chunging exercise so important? Following are my observations of two currently popular types of exercises. One, fast aerobic exercise, is promoted by a famous movie actress through video tapes. The other, slow bending and stretching exercise like yoga, is promoted by another beautiful lady on television. And they have both been doing this for years. Nevertheless, when you compare their appearance to five years ago, they certainly look older now than before.

Why, with all their efforts, are these two women still aging? I believe that fast exercise is *too* fast and *too* jarring, which damages and ages the internal body. And when I watch the breathing techniques of the yoga instructor, I see that she uses chest breathing over abdominal breathing, and her stretching is unnatural.

It is a proven fact that the appearance and movement of the human body are able to be improved until the age of seventy by proper exercise. Scientists have noticed that a well-fit person at age seventy is stronger, faster and in much better shape than an unfit person at thirty years of age.

At age sixty-nine, a man who has a difficult time walking even one block, if determined to improve his physical abilities, can work toward that goal every day. By the time he reaches the age of seventy, he can walk two or three blocks with ease. In all likelihood, he will also appear younger, feel better, and be more energetic.

During the years in which I was developing the Chunging exercises, I noticed myself become stronger and faster. My appearance actually looked younger. I became rejuvenated. My patients and friends noticed the difference. They say I have tapped the fountain of youth!

I am confident that I will be more physically and mentally functional when I reach age 70 than I was at age 30 if I am able to continue my good behavior and keep up my Chunging exercises.

Gastro-Intestinal Chunging

A typical and misguided approach to gastro-intestinal problems is the immediate taking of over-the-counter or prescription drugs for common symptoms such as nausea, vomiting, and diarrhea.

I have seen patients taking anti-nausea drugs for obvious food poisoning. The quickest cure for food poisoning is to vomit and eliminate the cause, the poisoned food, and get it out of the gut as completely and as soon as possible. Food poisoning is real poisoning in that the body is being attacked by toxins produced by bacteria in contaminated food.

By suppressing the first mechanism (the nausea which is alerting you to the problem), you prolong the poisoning. If you take something to keep you from vomiting, the toxins have that much longer to work on your system, making you much sicker than you would have been if you had just thrown up as soon as you first felt like it. Headaches, weakness, and diarrhea are much more likely to develop due to the delay caused by not vomiting when you should have.

Diarrhea

When it comes to cleansing the body of toxins, diarrhea is the same as vomiting. They are both part of your body's natural disease fighting mechanism. Diarrhea develops when the bowels need to get rid of their contents as soon as possible.

As inconvenient as it may be, please just let the body's natural healing mechanism do its job. Let the feces go out, as nature intended. At least for a day or two, don't inhibit the process by taking medication to stop diarrhea. Your body really needs to clear out the system for one reason or another. Try to determine the cause, so you can avoid it in the future.

Then, let your bowels rest by skipping the next regular meal. When the mealtime after that comes around, whether or not you still have diarrhea, eat only diluted rice soup (any brand of rice soup diluted four times with water then boiled ten minutes). Diarrhea will stop in less than 24 hours. Retaining toxic feces with medication only makes you sicker longer.

Causes of Most Abdominal Problems

Most abdominal problems are due to one or more of three simple causes.

1. Constipation.

2. Eating too much food.

3. Ingesting contaminated food.

How Constipation Develops

Every healthy infant has a bowel movement soon after each meal. This is normal. However, when the child becomes toilet trained, he learns that if he soils his underwear, his parents will be disappointed. To keep his parents happy, the child will attempt to hold his waste, which may end in constipation. I believe female children have a greater tendency to develop constipation than males because girls seem to try to please their parents more than boys. This may be one reason there are more constipated women than men.

People who move their bowels only when they have the urge to will most likely develop constipation. This is a bad habit. The only way to protect yourself against constipation for your entire life is to form the habit of moving your bowels regularly.

Bowel habits are just that—*habits.* Fortunately, habits can be changed, no matter how old you are at the time you begin to change your habits.

When you do have the urge to evacuate your bowels, don't wait. Conversely, when you don't have the urge to move your bowels but you know you should, stimulate them with Chunging exercises.

There are hundreds of medicines that you can take to treat constipation. However, none of these drugs will eliminate constipation for your entire life. Learning and practicing better bowel habits will avoid the many dangerous and disgusting problems associated with long term constipation.

How to Prevent and Eliminate Constipation

The usual waste products from food intake should be well-formed, that is, the stool should be neither too hard nor too soft. A diet with enough fiber gives the intestines something to push along, something to brush up the waste products, so to speak. Water is the partner of fiber in performing this task. The bowels, like the kidneys, need water to do their work.

Feces have three components, which are:

1. Undigested food (part of which could be toxic).

2. Germs in the colon, some of which may aid in digestion, but which also produce toxic chemicals.

3. Secretions from the pancreas, liver, and intestines, which aid digestion but which are toxic if reintroduced to the body.

As you can see from this description, all three components of feces contain toxic chemicals. If you don't remove these chemicals regularly, at least once a day, your cells will be slowly poisoned in a way that will inevitably lead to disease.

I know there are many doctors who say that everyone has their own individual bowel habits. They claim that even if you move your bowels once every week you are normal. This is ridiculous! The accumulation of toxic chemicals universally leads to just one thing: disease. How can anyone consider constipation *normal*?

Chunging Exercise to Develop Good Bowel Habits

This exercise may seem rather silly, but if you continue practicing it every day, within six weeks you should have no more problems with constipation.

The following exercises will enable you to change bad bowel habits into healthful, invigorating good habits.

Step 1. At night, before you sleep, take some fiber in one of the over-the-counter brands of psylum in a recommended dosage with a glass of water.

Step 2. As soon as you awaken, drink one or two cups of water, preferably hot water.

Step 3. Sit on the toilet 15 to 20 minutes.

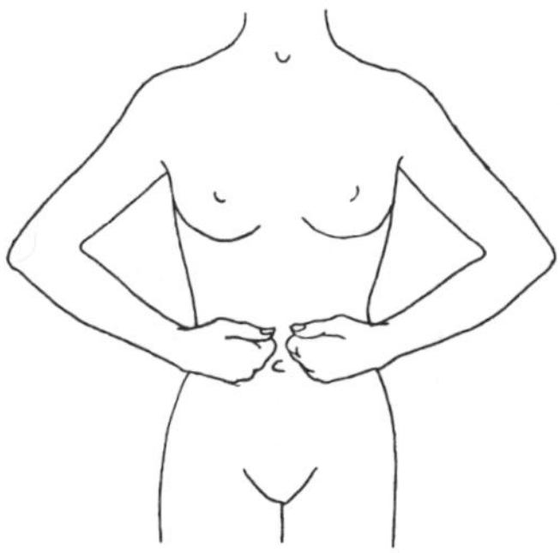

Step 4. Hold both fists together on the upper part of your abdomen. Then press gently inwards and roll your fists slowly down to your lower abdomen.

Step 5. Feel your entire abdomen with your fingertips. If you discover any points where there is discomfort or pain, rub those points until the pain disappears.

If you do not have a bowel movement within twenty minutes, do not worry. Simply repeat this exercise the next morning. If you wish to hasten the results of this exercise, you may take over-the-counter bowel softener every night until you develop good habitual bowel movements.

Chunging Exercises for the Intestines

The following exercises are meant to keep your abdominal organs healthy by promoting better circulation. These exercises are designed to be done every day—not only when you have a problem:

> Step 1. Rub your abdomen with your palms until your abdomen is warm.
>
> Step 2. Place your two fists in the middle of your upper abdomen. Pressing inwards and downwards, slowly move your fists to your pubis.
>
> Step 3. Place your two fists on both sides of your upper abdomen. Pressing inwards and downwards, roll your fists to your pubis.
>
> Step 4. Exhale through your mouth while you slowly roll your hands down to your lower abdomen. Then, inhale through your nose and repeat this procedure three to five times.

Please review Breath Chunging in the chapter on Breathing to perform this exercise correctly. This exercise promotes better flow of blood in the circulatory system of the bowel.

Live Longer by Eating Less

Of all the ideas which have been advanced for prolonging human functional life span, only one is almost universally agreed upon by the world's researchers. That idea is that the restriction of dietary intake does two things; it minimizes the frequency of disease and truly extends life span.

By reducing daily food intake to half of what they would eat if their diets were unrestricted, researchers can extend laboratory mammals' life-span 20 to 80 percent and also reduce all kinds of disease by 50%.

The same thing is true of people. Well-nourished but underfed humans live longer and are more functional until death.

The fundamental cause of aging and disease is the malfunction of body cells, induced mainly by poisonous chemicals from external and internal sources. External poisons are ingested daily as a food. No food is completely free from harsh ingredients that can harm cells. Even chemicals like iodine and potassium, which are essential for human life, can harm a person when ingested in excess.

Since excess food acts as poison to living cells, a person who eats less will encounter less disease. Please remember that one more spoonful of food fed to a child after an adequate meal is a spoonful of potential problems. One extra bite after a proper meal is like a drop of poisonous waste to your body.

In primitive times, humans could not predict the time of their next meal. They had to eat a lot when there was food to prepare for a possible period of famine. A person today who satisfies his appetite eats double of what is needed. This is especially true of an overweight person.

Americans tend to stuff themselves and their children. The result is that 75 % of our population are overweight at present. Over the last fifty years, Americans have become fatter every year, and are expected to get fatter in future.

Most Americans could benefit by reducing their amount of food intake by half. By this, I don't mean dieting. I mean to actually stop eating before you are full—every day.

Overeating is a conditioned reflex formed by eating habits in early life. I often hear a mother proudly tell me that her child, who I delivered six months ago, is now the same weight as her neighbor's one-year-old. She thinks having a plump baby proves she is a good mother. However, children who are fatter through infancy and childhood become overweight adults. Do not damn your child by overfeeding in the name of love.

Please do develop the following good habits:

1. Chew well before you swallow.

2. Stop eating before full.

3. Move your bowels every day.

If you develop these good habits and eat less, you will almost never suffer from GI problems. If you raise your children to have these three good habits in their early life, your children will be blessed with long and healthy life.

A large amount food is harder to pass through the channel of the intestines. The action that moves food through the bowels is called peristalsis (the rhythmic movement of the intestines). If the body has to work hard to move the feces along, the result may be severe cramps. Abnormal peristalsis is the cause of the four cardinal symptoms of GI disturbance: abdominal pain, nausea, vomiting, and diarrhea.

The large volume of accumulated feces will also weaken the muscular walls of your bowels, which will result in diverticulosis and diverticulitis. A person who has daily, regular bowel movements will usually not be afflicted with these diseases

Prevent and Eliminate Fecal Incontinence

Fecal incontinence is a spontaneous, uncontrolled bowel movement, which can happen any time, any place. Fecal incontinence develops for approximately one out of five people by the age of sixty-nine, and one out of every three by the age of seventy-nine. This unpleasant condition can often (but not always) be eliminated by following a simple set of Chunging exercises.

I suggest that you begin my Perianal Chunging exercises (on the following page), and continue this easy muscle-toning exercise for the rest of your life. Almost all people, both men and women, who do this Perianal Chunging exercise regularly, succeed in accomplishing its goals. If you avoid the miserable problems that come with incontinence in later years, old age will not be so difficult. You will avoid frustration and embarrassment, and you will save a lot of money.

Perianal Chunging

Perianal Chunging is a type of Breath Chunging.

> Step 1. Exhale through your mouth slowly. Then simply close your mouth, and automatically inhale. Only your lower abdomen should expand on inhaling.
>
> Step 2. As soon as you are finished inhaling, hold your breath and constrict your anal sphincter as tightly as possible as you count to five. Exhale through your mouth again and repeat the first step. Continue these two Perianal Chunging steps at least 20 times every day for the rest of your life.

Like other muscles, the anal sphincter needs to be regularly exercised. Not only will this exercise prevent or cure fecal incontinence, but you will see other benefits as well. For instance, regular Perianal Chunging will keep you calmer and lower your blood pressure. If you suffer from headaches, they will lessen. If you are impotent, your erections will be stiffer and last longer.

If you are already suffering from fecal incontinence or diarrhea, this exercise will be worth a million dollars. I know what a frightening and uncomfortable experience incontinence can be, because I, myself, experienced this and now have cured incontinence with my Perianal Exercise.

If you have not yet experienced incontinence, please *do not disregard these exercises.* Remember, there is a fifty percent chance that someday you will be afflicted with either fecal or urinary incontinence or both. Urinary incontinence is discussed in the following chapter.

The goal of Chunging is to remain fully functional; a fully functional person is not incontinent. I assure you that if you practice my Perianal exercise daily, you will improve your ability to control your bowels. A good time to practice this exercise is when driving a car or watching television, or any time you have a few minutes alone. Do Perianal Chunging regularly. Do it! It is important!

External Hemorrhoids

An external hemorrhoid is an inflammation and infection of a vein around the anus due to the presence of a thrombus (blood clot) in the vein. It is called external because it forms outside of the body, in the blood vessels near the surface and around the outside of the anus, not inside the rectum where regular hemorrhoids form.

An external hemorrhoid can range from uncomfortable to downright painful. Simple surgery may be required. The most common causes of external hemorrhoids are liver disease, chronic constipation, chronic diarrhea, and pregnancy.

Blood is more heavily supplied to the anus than to most other portions of the body. Also, the veins around the anus are close to the surface of the skin. Since soap washes away the protective oil of the skin, germs from the anus can easily infect the skin, causing inflammation. Since anal veins are so close to the skin, the walls of the veins can also get inflamed and swell, narrowing the veins, and causing slower venous blood flow. These two factors, inflammation of the vein walls and slower venous flow, create an environment in which blood clots easily develop. The blood clot expands the size of the vein, until finally, if untreated, the vein ruptures and bleeds.

If you stop using soap, this vicious cycle will stop, and your external hemorrhoids will disappear within one year.

Bladder and Kidney

A normal, healthy adult produces approximately 2,000 cc of urine every day. The normal capacity of the urinary bladder is between 200 and 300 cc's. This means that you must urinate seven to ten times every day in order to keep your bladder healthy.

There are people who brag that they urinate only two or three times a day. These people are distending their bladders two to four times beyond their normal capacity. This weakens their bladder muscles, which makes them unable to expel all the urine in their bladders when they urinate. Residual urine left in the bladder is frequently the source of bladder infections. Try to empty your bladder every two hours when you are awake.

By the time you are eighty, there is almost a 50% chance that you will be afflicted by either fecal or urinary incontinence. There is a great deal you can do to increase your chances of remaining in the group which does not have these dreadful problems. The time to start preventive maintenance is now!

Kidney Chunging

To keep your kidneys and bladder functional all your life, follow these simple suggestions:

- Don't drink soft drinks. Anyone with kidney or bladder problems should not drink carbonated beverages. Soft drinks change the normal pH of urine. In time, this will weaken both the kidneys and bladder, causing disease.

- Drink plenty of water to flush waste and germs from the kidneys and bladder.

- Do the following Kidney Chunging exercises:

  Step 1. Place your palms over the area of both kidneys and rub until that area feels warm.

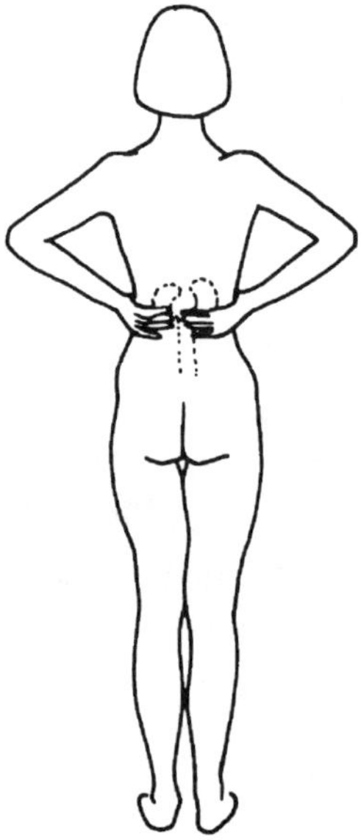

Step. 2. Place your hands in a V-shape over your sacrum (middle of your lower back) and rub until it is warm.

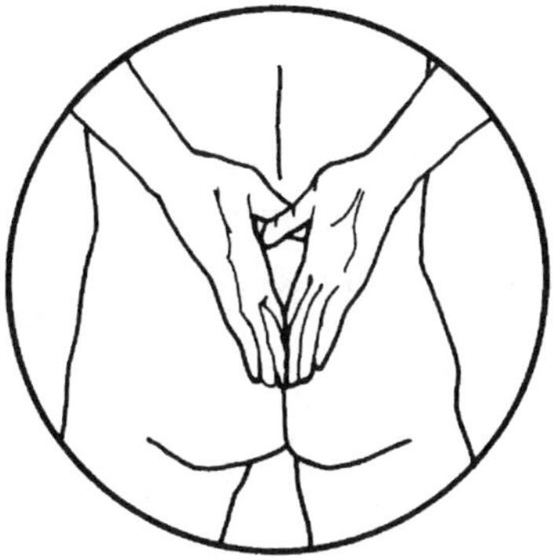

Kidney Chunging exercises increase circulation to the kidney area. Increased circulation will help people with chronic kidney problems such as infections, kidney stones and hypertension. If you are fortunate enough not to have those problems, these exercises will help prevent them.

Prevent and Eliminate Urinary Incontinence

Urinary incontinence is one of the major afflictions of women of old age. Urination is controlled by complex neuro-muscular functions. For the elderly, the loss of muscle tone, merely as a consequence of aging, is a very difficult problem. Loss of control of the bladder sphincter is one of the most embarrassing and socially inhibiting conditions which may develop with aging. Urinary incontinence is common in women over the age of forty, but is infrequent in men.

Kegel Exercises

Arnold H. Kegel, M.D., invented a simple exercise which prevents or cures urinary incontinence in women, as well as having other beneficial muscle toning effects.

Since incontinence is so stressful and the cost of adult diapers is so high, I am surprised that more women with this problem don't control their incontinence with Kegel exercises.

I strongly recommend that every women over forty follow these directions and faithfully do this easy exercise every day for the rest of her life.

How to Learn the Kegel Exercise

These instructions are, of course, for women:

1. When you urinate, become aware of which muscles start and stop the flow of urine.

2. While urinating (at a time when you have an average volume of urine in your bladder), practice starting and stopping the flow. If you try this when you have to go, due to an unusually large volume of urine, it won't be as successful as with a smaller volume. Concentrate on learning which muscles you are using to stop the flow.

3. Practice using the same muscles when you are not urinating. Tighten the muscles as tight as you can,

then relax completely. *That is all there is to it.* At first, try to do this 35 times. You may find it tiring to even do that many when you first begin these exercises. It will get easier with practice in just a few days.

5. The next day, increase the number by 5, and continue increasing by 5 every day until you can do 50 without feeling tired.

6. Do the exercises in sets; do 4 sets of 50 with a rest in between, every day. In other words, 200 a day will keep the muscles which control the flow of urine, toned and in good working order. More is better.

7. The Kegel exercises can be done from any position, sitting, standing, or lying down. They don't all have to be done at one time. Do 100 in the morning, 100 when you are watching TV, or waiting for a bus.

Kegel Chunging

When you have mastered the Kegel Exercise, combine at least half of your Kegel muscle tightenings with Breath Chunging:

Step 1. Exhale slowly through your mouth. Then close your mouth, and you will automatically inhale. Your chest wall should not expand; only your abdomen should move.

Step 2. As soon as you have finished inhaling, hold your breath and constrict the urinary sphincter as tightly as possible and keep it contracted as you slowly exhale through your mouth. For an explanation, see the chapter on Breath Chunging.

If you do not have an incontinence problem, wonderful. You positively need to do these exercises to keep yourself in shape. We are dealing with muscle tone here; use it or lose it.

If you do already have a slight problem, such as leaking a few drops of urine when you laugh or cough, Kegel Chunging exercises will stop the problem in a few weeks.

If you don't do the exercises, the problem will become worse and worse. If you do the Kegel exercises for a while, and the problem stops, it will return if you let your muscle tone slacken. You *must* keep doing them .

If you are doing the Kegel exercises, and the problem returns, you are probably not squeezing the muscles hard enough or keeping the muscles taut long enough. Try that for a few weeks. You really can't cheat. If you neglect the exercises, skip a few days, and are casual about how hard you try, incontinence will return. However, if you have really worked hard at your Kegel exercises and the problem persists, see a urologist or gynecologist. There *are* surgical solutions to the problem, but obviously avoiding surgery by exercise is by far the better course of action.

The sphincter muscles are, after all, just muscles. Muscles respond to being used. No matter how flabby a set of muscles may have gotten, they can be toned up by working those muscles. If you have tried Kegel exercises before and failed, try again. Put some effort into it. Success in this area of your body is well worth the effort.

Common Skin Diseases

The three most common skin diseases—acne, psoriasis, and eczema—cause discomfort, embarrassment, and expensive medical bills. They can be controlled by following these Skin Chunging exercises.

Acne

Acne is an inflammation caused by the blockage of sebaceous (oil) ducts. If germs are introduced to this system, an abscess is formed. There are two reasons for the development of acne:

1. An overproduction of oil
2. A blockage of oil ducts.

The purpose of body oil is to protect our skin tissue. However, humans frequently wash this kind friend away with soap. In order to compensate for this depletion, the skin *increases* its production of oil.

Oil production glands have a small hole (duct) that allows only a normal amount of oil to flow. If there is an overproduction of oil due to soap stimulation, this hole will become blocked since it cannot accommodate such large quantities of oil. The blockage that occurs inevitably leads to inflammation (acne).

Let's follow the development of acne through the case of one of my patients, Alex. When Alex was twelve, she washed her face only once each day, sometimes missing a day. Also, she used as little soap as possible because it burned her eyes.

When she turned thirteen, Alex became more aware of her appearance, so she began to use soap daily to wash her face. Then she began washing her face with soap twice a day. For a while, she looked cleaner and healthier than before. However, after six months, some pimples appeared. (It usually takes six months of soap stimulation to substantially increase the production of oil.)

Of course, wishing to eliminate her pimples, she started applying stronger soap to her face three to five times a day. However, since increasing the use of soap only increases the amount of oil production, her acne became worse. After a year, the acne had spread all over her face.

Alex finally went to see her family doctor who advised her to use over-the-counter acne products. This doctor honestly believed that these medications would help her skin eruptions; however, Alex found that her problem progressed to the point where abscesses were forming under the skin. A dermatologist then gave Alex antibiotics to suppress her infections and abscesses. The dermatologist also gave her cleansing cream and special facial soap. Alexandra's acne problem seemed to be getting better for awhile. Whenever she went off her medication, her acne would become much worse. So, she went to the dermatologist every three to six months for more medication until she was twenty-seven. By this time, the excessive passage of oil through the oil ducts had dilated the ducts to the point of visibility. (The pores had become enlarged.) Although less acne developed, the widened ducts made her skin resemble an orange peel.

That dermatologist went through four years of college, four years of medical school, and four more years of residency to learn how to treat diseases.

To truly cure a disease, one must eliminate the source of the disease.

Alexandra's dermatologist did exactly what he learned in medical school. He treated the symptoms of her acne problem without eliminating the cause of the acne. With treatment of this type, the disease never goes away. It merely becomes tolerable. The medicine that the dermatologist gave Alexandra successfully combated the symptoms of her acne problem by widening the passage so that oil could flow easily and by fighting the infections with antibiotics.

Why didn't the dermatologist ever think to advise his patient to stop stimulating the production of oil? If the dermatologist had advised her to stop using soap, and to start cleaning her face gently with water only, and to rub it only with her hands and not with a wash cloth, she could have been really cured within three years—without the scarring that occurred.

Psoriasis

Although psoriasis is not infectious, it is a fairly common skin disease. People shy away from patients who have a bad case, due to the presence of awful-looking lesions all over their bodies.

People with psoriasis feel dirty because of the red, scaly, swollen, oozing patches on their skin.

Dermatologists tell patients that psoriasis is an incurable disease and give patients who are afflicted with this problem some type of cortisone product. This temporarily eliminates the symptoms. The psoriasis seems to subside for a while, but after discontinuing the medication, the psoriasis rapidly reappears.

I believe the answer is very simple. Chemical pollutants applied to the surface of the skin are the cause of psoriasis. If a patient with psoriasis discontinues the use of soap, and begins Skin Chunging, it is very likely that his disease will disappear. At the very least, it will not get worse. (If you have psoriasis and still have it one year after you have discontinued the use of soap, please follow *all* the instructions I give in this book for general health.)

When people have even a mild skin problem, they tend to wash more often, wash longer, and use more and stronger soaps. Skin problems make people feel icky, and it is a natural reaction to want to wash the problem away. This extra washing certainly increases the irritation instead of diminishing it. It prevents the skin's natural defenses from having a chance to do their job. It comes down to the soap damaging individual skin cells, and as a result, the cells' inability to function correctly.

When germs or chemical irritants attempt to enter your body through your skin, your skin begins to attack these intruders, sending more blood to the skin, which causes it to become reddish. Your skin then sends nerve impulses to the brain which in turn sends back the sensation of itching or burning of the affected area, in order to draw your attention to the germ's or poison's attack. Itching makes you want to do something about it, to scratch. If your skin feels hot and inflamed, you want to do something about that, too. Your instinct for patting cool water on the irritated spot is very primitive—and very correct.

Cortisone products work chiefly by halting the body's normal defense mechanism. When infection is present, more blood gallops to the rescue at that spot. But cortisone suppresses the defense mechanism. Thus, treatment with cortisone misleads the body into thinking there is no disease or irritant, and because cortisone represses the system, even less blood comes to the lesion. No nerve impulses are then sent to the brain saying there is a problem, as no irritation or itching is felt. Cortisone has tricked the immune system. Most skin disease symptoms—rashes, itching, and irritation—go away temporarily after treatment with cortisone, but the diseases are not cured.

Persistent chemical poisoning makes skin cells act abnormally, thus causing skin diseases like moles or skin cancer. You can safely assume that most common skin diseases were induced by the abuse of soap.

Eczema

Skin cells can still fight germs even if they are not completely dead; however, the dying skin cells cannot do the job effectively, as they have been poisoned with soap.

That attracts more blood to the area which makes the skin turn red. White blood cells start killing germs, and a pussy discharge is formed. The skin becomes irritated and itchy. This is called eczema.

When eczema starts bothering older people, they think they are allergic or sensitive to soap and stop using soap. They wash with water only, but don't tell anyone; they are afraid people will start accusing them of smelling bad. After a time, the eczema disappears, and their skin starts living again. Living skin has the power to kill germs. Germs can't live on healthy, living skin.

A few older adults realize the harmful effects of soap. They only wash their skin with water, which keeps their skin alive and disease-free.

Living Skin

Babies' skin is very soft and smells good after their baths even without perfumed soaps or powders. Why? Babies' skin has a pleasant smell because the skin cells are all alive. Living skin has a good, clean, 'living' smell. A year after you begin Skin Chunging, your skin, too, will be alive and disease-free.

The American Perception of Medicine

Two health-related topics about which I can easily agree with popular opinion is that health care in America is too expensive and that the health care system needs to be changed.

However, I see a much different health care crisis in America than most Americans perceive.

The American health care system is ill. Like any human disease, this illness has factors which cause the problems. If the causes were eliminated, the crisis in health care would soon disappear.

Unfortunately, just as well-respected American doctors approach medicine from the supply side, most of the politicians, Democrat or Republican, address only the symptoms of the crisis. They present all kinds of ideas to ease the severity of the crisis rather than finding the causes of the crisis and eliminating them.

By studying the history of Communism, I see two major causes of its failure, and I believe the same two causes will defeat the present health plan and any future health care plans. These are the same factors which have doomed many great government plans throughout history:

1. Abusers eventually overburdened the systems.

2. The basic philosophies upon which the plans were based were not in tune with human nature.

First, let's address the three major abusers of the American health care system.

1. The public has a wrong perception of what constitutes good medical care.

2. Doctors who do *not* cure their patients are rewarded financially more than those who do cure patients.

3. The present legal system forces physicians to practice defensive medicine.

The Public's Wrong Perception of Good Medical Care

Most people feel that they had good medical care when they received expensive medicine after numerous expensive tests. Many patients feel neglected and even angry when doctors don't give them drugs and tests, or if they receive less expensive medicines or few tests.

Even if their disease gets worse, they like to think "my doctor did everything he could do for my mysterious, rare disease."

If they get better or are cured of disease, they are not necessarily comfortable; they think the doctor may have missed finding a serious problem because he did not perform all the tests, especially extremely complicated tests. In fact, more than half of all human illnesses can be cured with few or no drugs and without testing.

The Public's Ignorance of the Real Relationship Between Behavior and Disease

There is a very real cause and effect between bad behavior and poor health.

Non-smokers have finally figured this out and for the first time have begun to take action by demanding smoke-free restaurants and offices. Mothers Against Drunk Driving has been effective in decreasing the horrible injuries and fatalities caused by irresponsible drunken behavior. The public is more aware of the relationship between a fatty diet and various health problems like heart attacks, high blood pressure, and breast cancer. But those are just a few of many bad habits which have a direct adverse effect on health—and which therefore affect the cost of health care.

There needs to be massive re-learning of simpler, cleaner lifestyles. Television could do this. Schools *should* do this. Hospitals, insurance companies, ad agencies, everyone should promote this idea. The public image of health care needs to be personalized; only *you* can keep yourself healthy. Your body is *your* responsibility. There *is* a relationship between good behavior and good health. No health care system can do it for you if you won't do it for yourself.

Reward Doctors for Health, Not Illness

Doctors who do *not* cure the disease are rewarded by multiple visits of patients. This encourages prolonging the illness or at least discourages curing it so fast. With each office visit by the patient, the doctor gains profit. But the present health care system offers little monetary reward for being a good healer.

For example, many early cases of hypertension and adult diabetes get better by proper diet and exercise. Chronic sinusitis can be cured by proper nose cleansing. Recurrent vaginitis can be prevented and eliminated by simply stopping the use of soap when washing.

There are very few doctors who just prescribe good behavior, such as diet and exercise, before putting their patient on drugs only. The current trend has been to write prescriptions for a thirty day supply of medicine or less, even if the patient really needs to take the medicine on a continuing basis. The patients of the 'pill pushers' have to keep visiting their doctor's office for more prescriptions, and soon those patients develop side effects from the medicine and the severity of the disease increases. Instead of getting well, the patients become sicker, requiring even greater expense.

Stop Forcing Physicians to Practice Defensive Medicine

I really believe that the American concept, 'all people are equal under the law', is a universal holy law which will eventually come to be adopted by all nations. Occasionally, however, this fair and just view of law is filtered through the American legal system in such a way that the results become twisted through the lawyers' legal antics.

There is no equity between judgments in similar cases tried by different judges and by different juries. By breaking this equality of American law, they say justice is done. We all hear stories about malpractice law suits against physicians which, for instance, award a crippled infant sixty million dollars while another jury may award only one hundred thousand dollars for a similar crippling injury to another child caused by a drunken driver. What a discrepancy!

The lawyer then takes half of that poor (now rich), crippled infant's money as his fee. Enormous legal fees like this give plenty of incentive for attorneys to seek multimillion dollar settlements. Because of this, the legal profession blocks any attempts by lawmakers to make malpractice awards more equal. Probably every lawyer dreams of the 'one big case' out there which will make him a rich man. They are practicing jury lottery, not justice.

After a lifetime of work, most physicians' whole life savings are just a small fraction of the sixty million dollars. A thirty million dollar payment to the lawyer for a single case is too much. This is robbery, not justice. I hope juries know that in the long run all of this award money comes from patients, not from the doctor or insurance company.

Fear of this type of big award induces the doctor to practice defensive medicine on every single patient he attends, which is a tremendous cost burden on the entire health care system of this country. Defensive medicine means that in order to protect themselves against possible future lawsuits, the doctors must order totally unnecessary tests—just to be able to prove, in case that patient ever takes them to court, that all possibilities were considered. What a ridiculous financial drain this is on the entire economy!

The greatest abusers of our health care system are not the welfare mothers who may unnecessarily take their children to the emergency room, but those greedy malpractice lawyers and, I'm sorry to say, those gullible juries.

The President Clinton, or his successor, will continue to consult with experts from all fields of medicine. In all likelihood, more governmental health plans will be presented amidst claims that they will work.

People already know the results of these plans. They would probably work in a cumbersome way, but would also be expensive to manage, be far less efficient than the minimally controlled system we have had in the past, and would provide people with lower quality health care. We have witnessed the results of the experiences of other countries along these lines.

Why did the old plans fail? Why will the new plan fail? Because they are looking for solutions in the wrong places. It is not the fault of the health care delivery system, which, in America, could and should be excellent.

The fault is in the philosophy behind modern conventional medicine. I believe the basic approach to resolving medical problems is totally backwards. Treating the symptoms does not cure the disease. You have a headache? Take an aspirin! Does that address the cause of the headache or prevent headaches or cure headaches? It does not. It is the *cause* that should be investigated and eliminated. Prescribing drugs to relieve the symptoms so the patient can get back to work as soon as possible, making him *feel* he is better, is what I call the Supply Side of Medicine.

The Supply Side of Medicine is Wrong

The basic philosophy behind any system must be in tune with human nature in order to be successful and to last a long time.

Conventional American medicine concentrates too much on the development of miracle drugs to fight diseases. I believe that finding better drugs may actually be among the least important factors in achieving better health.

Almost every week pharmaceutical companies create another drug which has a longer list of side effects than it does beneficial effects. Men and women of medicine stand ready to give patients all kinds of treatments, through all the entrances of the human body.

I call this practice the 'Supply Side of Medicine'. Sometimes, we see good results from the conventional supply side of medicine. The incapacitating symptoms become tolerable to the patient and the disease becomes weaker and often disappears when the patient receives that treatment. Soon, however, the beneficial effects of the treatment are gone. The symptoms return because the disease has not been cured even though the symptoms disappeared for a while. And so the symptoms slowly get worse and the disease gets harder and harder to treat. Problems arise from side effects of the drugs used in the treatment. Conventional medicine almost never really cures a disease because it is treating the symptoms instead of cleansing away the cause of disease.

Switch Medical Thinking to the Cleansing Side of Medicine

Only the elimination of the cause of the disease will cure or prevent disease. I call this view of health care the 'Cleansing Side of Medicine'.

Step by step in this book, I have tried to present my beliefs and show you how, by Chunging, you can get yourself back in shape. What can be done on a personal basis can *and should* be done nationally to improve the entire health care system. The American medical community must change:

- Switch from Supply Side thinking to the Cleansing Side of Medicine.

- Direct medical attention and research to cause-finding rather than to symptom treating or 'cover-ups'.

- American medical schools must teach doctors to listen to their patients and to ask them 'why'.

- Change the malpractice laws from state to national—and force Congress to use common sense.

- Educate people in early school years about such mundane topics as proper bowel habits, the importance of breathing clean air, and drinking plenty of water.

We must develop the attitude of searching for the cause of disease. We must ask ourselves "What did I do wrong, what did I do differently today to bring on this headache?" We should direct our thinking to this line of thought: "How could I eliminate the cause of this headache so I can cure the headache and prevent its future recurrence?" Until most of us, patients and physicians alike, develop this attitude, the American health care crisis will not be solved.

Adults resist efforts to make them change their behavior. Only a real understanding of the wonderful, beneficial effects of good behavior will make them want to give up their favorite bad behavior habits. To a great extent, they already know in their hearts that what I have said in this book is true. It will take a great public relations campaign to actually make them mend their ways.

If you have read this book, it is my hope that you will take my ideas to heart, and use the cleansing Chunging Exercises to improve the quality of your own life.

The human body could and should be in perfect health, free of disease, if it is clean inside and out, free of toxic wastes. A clean body can achieve perfect harmony. After all, man is made in the image of God. Man is made to be perfect.

Index